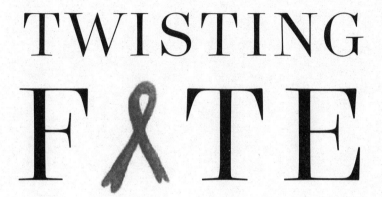

TWISTING FATE

TWISTING
FTE

MY JOURNEY *with* BRCA— *from* BREAST CANCER DOCTOR *to* PATIENT *and* BACK

PAMELA N. MUNSTER, MD

THE EXPERIMENT

NEW YORK

The Experiment, LLC
220 East 23rd Street, Suite 600, New York, NY 10010-4658
theexperimentpublishing.com

This book contains the opinions and ideas of its author. It is intended to provide helpful and informative material on the subjects addressed in the book. It is sold with the understanding that the author and publisher are not engaged in rendering medical, health, or any other kind of personal professional services in the book. The author and publisher specifically disclaim all responsibility for any liability, loss, or risk—personal or otherwise—that is incurred as a consequence, directly or indirectly, of the use and application of any of the contents of this book.

Many of the designations used by manufacturers and sellers to distinguish their products are claimed as trademarks. Where those designations appear in this book and The Experiment was aware of a trademark claim, the designations have been capitalized.

The Experiment's books are available at special discounts when purchased in bulk for premiums and sales promotions as well as for fund-raising or educational use. For details, contact us at info@theexperimentpublishing.com.

Library of Congress Cataloging-in-Publication Data

Names: Munster, Pamela N., author.
Title: Twisting fate : my journey with BRCA—from breast cancer doctor to patient and back / Pamela N. Munster, MD
Description: New York : The Experiment, [2018]
Identifiers: LCCN 2018020072 (print) | LCCN 2018031477 (ebook) | ISBN 9781615195145 (ebook) | ISBN 9781615194780 (cloth)
Subjects: LCSH: Munster, Pamela N.—Health. | Breast—Cancer—Patients—Biography. | Women physicians—Biography. | Breast—Cancer—Treatment.
Classification: LCC RC280.B6 (ebook) | LCC RC280.B6 M86 2018 (print) | DDC 362.19699/4490092 [B]—dc23
LC record available at https://lccn.loc.gov/2018020072

ISBN 978-1-61519-478-0
Ebook ISBN 978-1-61519-514-5

Text and cover design by Sarah Smith
Author photograph by Nicola Pitaro

Manufactured in the United States of America

First printing September 2018
10 9 8 7 6 5 4 3 2 1

Contents

Chapter 1: **An Unexpected Call:** Screening and Diagnosing Breast Cancer   1

Chapter 2: **Mastectomy, Still Needed?** Surgical Approaches to Breast Cancer   23

Chapter 3: **Reconstruction:** Surgical Options and Decisions   45

Chapter 4: **Adjuvant Therapy for Breast Cancer:** Why Early Detection Is Important   63

Chapter 5: **The Day Before:** Preparing for Breast Cancer Surgery   89

Chapter 6: **The Day Of**   101

Chapter 7: **Hereditary Cancer and BRCA Mutations:** Preventing Ovarian Cancer   123

Chapter 8: **Prostate Cancer:** BRCA Mutations Don't Spare Men   151

Chapter 9: **Back to Normal:** Feeling, and Fighting, the Cancer Blues   163

Chapter 10: **Curse or Cure?** My Dad's BRCA-Related Pancreatic Cancer Story   181

Chapter 11: **Life After Lis:** How a Family Copes with Loss   201

Chapter 12: **The Gift of BRCA:** Getting Tested for Cancer Mutations   229

Afterword   255

Acknowledgments   259

About the Author   263

Chapter 1

An Unexpected Call:
Screening and Diagnosing Breast Cancer

I t was just before my twentieth birthday and I was back home for Carnival in Vilters, Switzerland. Our entire village had come out to celebrate the time before Lent until the wee hours of the morning. It was an exciting time: I was a first-year medical student and a gorgeous associate history professor had finally asked me out back at school in Berne, after a year of hopeful waiting for this date. I danced with my old high school friends all through the night and without any sleep went skiing the next morning. By late afternoon, I was exhausted and wanted to get to my parents' quickly. So rather than ride the gondola back down to the station, I took a shortcut across the top of a canyon to ski to their house. I probably was quite aware that it was risky to cross the ridge to get from one peak to the other, yet I felt invincible on skis and I had done this so many times.

About halfway along, I triggered an avalanche that caused me to plummet with the snow cloud 1,000 feet down. Somehow, I managed to stay afloat and came to a halt at the top of a cliff overlooking another thousand-foot drop.

Sitting there, chest-deep in the snow and looking over the edge, the first thing I did was panic. I looked back up the hill and it was terrifyingly steep. I'd had plenty of training from my years on the ski team, so I knew that hiking back up on an active avalanche field can trigger a second one. I panicked more. Then, almost as quickly, I felt a curious calm come over me. Everything was going to be fine. *This is no time to die*, I kept thinking. Not after I'd tried so hard to get that date.

Gingerly, I pulled myself out of the snowbank and inched my way up the hill through deep snow for what seemed like hours. I was barely halfway to the top when I was completely worn out and about to give up. It was sheer chance that the man running the ski lift had stepped out to take in the last rays of sunlight before closing up for the day. Looking out over the gully, he spotted me fighting my way up the mountain. He summoned another member of the ski patrol to come to my rescue. Steady and gently, the two men clipped me into a safety rope and then coaxed me to hike to the top of the hill, step by step, not looking at the snowfield ominously towering above me but down at my feet. Eventually we reached the snowmobile he had parked behind the ski patrol station and they got me down safely on the other side of the mountain.

Once home, my mother made me a hot chocolate and lit a fire. Exhausted and still shaken up, I was lying on the sofa when Dad called to ask why I wasn't at Carnival. Not really up for more dancing, I didn't even mention my harrowing ordeal, but mumbled something about being tired. Hours later, he came home furious—I was the talk of the town, this reckless girl who had skied across an avalanche field and had to be rescued by the lift operators.

The next morning I found him at the breakfast table, clearly still angry.

"You raised me to take risks and not to be afraid of everything," I said defiantly.

Completely still, he looked at me for a long time. Finally he said with a mixture of lingering worry and hidden pride, "Then go and conquer the world; just mind yourself!"

I gave him a hug and smiled at him, regaining my confidence. Two weeks later, I had my date with the gorgeous professor, instilling in me the confidence to keep going.

I learned then that often something good will come out of the most frightening of circumstances. This outlook on life is still with me today and has led me to establish a research center dedicated to learning about BRCA gene mutation and the risks of hereditary cancer.

But I'm getting ahead of myself . . .

Twenty-eight years later: I found myself having left my home country *and* the gorgeous professor to come to America and pursue a career in medical research. I was on a weekend ski trip in Montana. Sitting in a hot tub, I basked in the sun setting over the mountains. My girlfriends and I had just been talking about making plans for a future trip to Alaska when we all would turn fifty. Uncharacteristically for me, I was suddenly taken by a sense of doom and the thought *What if I'm not alive in two years?* I quickly brushed it off, turning my attention to the scenery around me. In that moment, out in the vast snowy mountains, with a wonderful family, great friends, and a fascinating career, life seemed all but perfect. But after returning back to San Francisco, the uneasy sense of something being amiss lingered.

I walked into my clinic at the University of California that Monday and was greeted by Tara, our nurse practitioner. Before she could hand me my schedule for the day's clinic, I interrupted her hastily to say, "Please schedule an appointment for a screening mammogram for me."

Taken clearly by surprise, she asked, "Why? You 'don't do' mammograms for somebody your age, especially without family history." And she was right; after a long discussion, our practice had settled on a unified approach in response to rapidly changing guidelines on mammograms, and decided not to screen women under the age of fifty. Which was the reason why I had not had a mammogram in seven years.

"Well, I feel I should have a mammogram. So please get me on the schedule before I change my mind," I replied with a shrug.

Tara just stared at me, but then nodded, a baffled look in her face. I could hear her mutter, "Whatever," rolling her eyes.

I can't explain why I went against my standard protocol of not screening women under fifty. Was it intuition? Regardless, something had triggered a gut decision; and even though I'm a scientist, I've *always* respected my instincts. And being a scientist has taught me that there is often more than we can explain.

Tara interrupted my thoughts, not letting the topic go: "Are you revisiting our approach to the current screening guidelines, after we finally settled on our recommendations, or is this an exception just for you?" she asked, genuinely curious.

"No, I just feel I should have a mammogram now," I repeated and, without further explanation, looked up the next patient's chart and focused on the person I was about to see.

Tara eyed me reflectively, and then said to my surprise: "I will order it immediately. Your instincts are usually right on."

Of course I order mammograms when they are indicated. A mammogram is an X-ray of the breast. It's a fast and relatively inexpensive test. Except there has been much confusion and debate in recent years about what is meant by *indicated* or *recommended*. Cancer experts and the major breast cancer societies, including the American Cancer Society (ACS), American College of Radiology (ACR), American Society of Clinical Oncology (ASCO), and the US Preventive Services Task Force (USPSTF) stage regular, heated debates on the topic, usually culminating in a further lack of consensus: just more evolving and contradictory recommendations on whom to screen, how often, and when to start and stop screening. There have been even more headlines in the media stating that mammograms could cause harm, leaving doctors and patients alike in a quandary on what is the best approach to breast cancer screening. These discussions on screening mammograms are centered on one fundamental question: Do routine screenings actually save lives? The answer is complicated: It does, but only for some women, not in general.

And here the debate goes deeper: What is the effectiveness of routine mammography screening in reducing both breast cancer–specific and overall mortality in the general population? And can the screening itself potentially cause physical and emotional harm?

There are probably no actual physical risks from having a mammogram, as the radiation exposure of mammograms is relatively small. There may be discomfort while the pictures are taken. However, having a test that may falsely diagnose cancer can lead to fears and unnecessary further imaging and breast biopsies.

Mammograms are our most commonly used screening tools for breast cancer; the first breast imaging was performed over one hundred years ago. In women without a suspected cancer, lump, or any changes in the breast or nipple, mammograms are done with the intent of *screening for cancer* and to detect *changes* in breast tissue that are suspicious.

In the screening mammograms, all women get the same set of pictures that are interpreted by a radiologist specifically trained in reading mammograms. The results are reported on a 6-point scale called the Breast Imaging Reporting and Data System (BI-RADS): 1 through 3 means normal, 4 and 5 are suspicious, and 6 is highly suggestive of cancer.

Routine screenings are based on the premise that the mammogram probably won't show any abnormality and that the radiologist is just screening the breast with no specific area to hone in on. The odds for accuracy are improved if the radiologist has a previous mammogram to see whether anything has changed.

In most cases, no suspicious areas are found, reported to the health care provider as BI-RADS 1–3, and the woman gets a letter in the mail stating that the mammogram was "normal" and to come back in one or two years. If the radiologist sees any suspicious areas or uncertainties, the patient will receive a phone call asking her to come back for more testing.

This sounds like it should be a pretty straightforward system easily employed for all women. So why should every woman not have a mammogram? Unfortunately, at present there are only clear recommendation for routine screenings (with an annual or biannual mammogram) established for women between ages of fifty and seventy-five. For the very young and older women, the recommendations are more controversial. There are several reasons to recommend against screening in women under fifty.

Ideally, the perfect screening tool would pick up with 100 percent certainty that an abnormality really is cancer and 100 percent certainty that if no abnormality is found, the test did not miss any cancer.

However, like most tests, mammograms are not perfect. The accuracy of detecting cancer depends upon the ability and experience of the radiologist to recognize suspicious changes in the breast and whether a cancer looks sufficiently different from the healthy tissue to be picked up. However, taken together, many larger studies suggest that screening mammograms on average detect true cancer only about 84 percent of the time. In actuality this means that not every woman who has an abnormal mammogram has cancer; very often she just needs to go back for more testing. Put into numbers from a specific study where over 400,000 women underwent screening mammograms, 112 in 1,000 women aged 40 to 49 had an abnormal mammogram but no cancer was later found on a repeat mammogram or a biopsy; compare this to the false positive rate of 70 in 1,000 in women over the age of 70. Detection is more precise in older women because they have more fatty tissue and fewer breast ducts, and breast cancer is more common in the average older women.

However, a normal mammogram doesn't necessarily mean that there is no cancer present, either—in the same study just discussed—one *true cancer* was missed in every thousand mammograms across all ages. Given how many mammograms are done every year, a large number of women will need extra tests due to a false positive mammogram and many cancers are missed in false negative mammograms.

Then why don't we instead use one of the more sophisticated technologies, such as breast MRI for screening young women? Unlike the mammogram's X-rays, an MRI uses a strong magnetic field. MRIs show much more detail than a mammogram. However, even more areas are picked up and considered suspicious, producing an even higher false positive rate. In average women under age fifty at low or average risk for breast cancer, there are thus many false positive findings. A false positive finding nonetheless requires follow-up scans and biopsies, just to confirm that no cancer is present.

Hence the most recent guidelines unanimously recommend regular screening with mammograms every year or two years for women between fifty and seventy-four. For younger women, some authorities recommend against it or at least impress on both women and health care providers to be mindful of false positives. For women seventy-five and older, recommendations will have to take in consideration other factors and overall health.

These guidelines are only applicable for women with average risk for breast cancer. For women at high risk for breast cancer, MRI and mammograms are both indicated and started much earlier in life, often even before a high-risk woman turns thirty.

When I ordered my own mammogram, I was at *low-risk* and thus fell under the more relaxed guidelines—"no screening necessary before age fifty." By these guidelines I should have waited with screening a bit longer, until I turned fifty. My last mammogram had been seven years prior, ordered by my obstetrician in Florida shortly after my daughter was born. But now there I was with my gut telling me that I should have a mammogram.

I went to have my mammogram a few days later. By the following Friday, I'd forgotten all about that impulsive decision. That weekend, I was out of town at a medical meeting, pouring myself a cup of coffee and talking with a colleague about a new research project testing a promising drug for advanced breast cancer. I can still remember the pulse and excitement of that day. It was a morning like many before—busy, hectic, and full of purpose.

I was just about to go back into the conference hall to hear the next presentation of new research data when my cell phone began to vibrate in my pocket. I almost didn't answer but then recognized the number of the university radiology department. The only reason its staff ever called me directly was with a "finding of concern." These days, such calls come only when there is bad news. The good news gets sent through the electronic chart system. With a pang of sadness, I mentally reviewed my recent patient list and pondered whom I'd have to subsequently call with bad news. Despite treating cancer patients for two decades, making such phone calls always feels like being in a real-life version of *The Hunger Games*.

The voice on the other end of the line sounded cheerful and upbeat. She told me that they had found five little "irregularities" on the March 15 scan, likely nothing of concern; I just needed to follow up.

Feeling distracted, I asked her what patient this was pertaining to—and she paused before saying, "Pamela, didn't you hear me? This is about *your* recent mammogram. We recommended a follow-up diagnostic mammogram for you."

That's when it hit me. She hadn't begun the conversation with her usual, "Hi, Dr. Munster, I'm calling with the CT or PET scan for . . ." She'd called me by my first name, as I did when following up with my patients, calling them with their news.

With a stabbing pain in my chest, I realized her call was meant for me. *My* mammogram was abnormal.

The voice on the other end of the phone said, "Please call the office to schedule your follow-up mammogram and don't forget to bring your previous mammograms so we can compare them. It is helpful to know whether any of these findings were there before."

It was Friday and I wouldn't be back at the clinic until the following Monday. A long time to wait for further scans and subsequent review, so my next phone call was to the radiology department at Moffitt Cancer Center in Tampa, my previous employer and health care provider. A friend and former colleague immediately left the phone to track down my early mammograms. She reported back that seven years ago the scans were normal, with no areas of concern, but given my current age, these old results didn't mean much.

I've made so many of those phone calls, sounding reassuring and upbeat—trying to soften the blow for patients, knowing full well that such calls never really reassure. I have spent many hours empathizing with the roller coaster of feelings that patients have when they learn of such scans and then have to wait days for results or further tests. I've always tried my best to be sensitive and understand what it must feel like to be in waiting; however, doctors are often so overwhelmed that there are many times when we don't get back to patients as quickly as we should.

Now here I was, trying to put in perspective what I just heard. Could this mean I had breast cancer? Breast cancer was a disease that I treated, not one that I should have. Ironically, of all the things I ever imagined having—and like all medical students, I had a lot of imagined diseases—breast cancer was just never one of them.

On that Friday morning, my "doctor" brain was confident that the likelihood of a breast cancer diagnosis was exceedingly low. All the statistics were very much in my favor. I repeated this in my mind, along with all the other positive indications: I couldn't feel a lump anywhere, and I know how to do a thorough physical exam. I was thin, athletic, didn't drink alcohol, and never used hormone supplements. I had had three pregnancies. Of all the risk factors associated with breast cancer, I had none.

That last one triggered my patient's brain and my own roller coaster began. Okay, I did have my first child when I was over age thirty; that's a risk factor. And I consume a lot of sugar.

Sugar, at least in rats, seems to be a risk factor for many illnesses, including cancer. I started repeating these additional facts in my head, over and over—dense breasts, so the mammogram was more likely to miss any cancer—a normal mammogram eight years ago may not have found a lump. But then, I did not feel a lump, so at worst the tumor would be small. And how many patients with big tumors have I seen who'd never felt a lump, either? I shook it off and tried reassuring myself that at my age, the false positive rate was really high. These findings likely meant nothing. That's what the radiology scheduler was really saying when asking me to return for more testing. Better be cautious—that is the process.

The chances of my having cancer were really minimal, but our emotions don't abide by cold probabilities. They usually conjure up the worst-case scenario instead. As on that day on the mountain, I was spiraling. There are, of course, those rare individuals with a more stoic disposition who can delay worrying until the bad facts are actually established. But I'm not one of those; it's just not in my nature. Weighing heavily into the reactions is the fact that every week, I care for patients whose breast cancer was not contained, and thus spread to other organs. Young women who die of this disease.

No matter how hard I tried reassuring myself, I couldn't win in the battle between my deep sense of knowing this was bad, and my numbers-driven medical brain telling me not to worry, that my risk for breast cancer was small. Those weren't just "little irregularities." I knew better. Not if there were five of them!

I had an endless weekend ahead, waiting to get another more complex mammogram to find out for sure. Of course, in the good moments of that weekend, I could briefly convince myself that in 112 of 1,000 abnormal mammograms in women my age, no cancer was eventually found.

The first thing Monday, I walked straight into radiology and asked for an appointment for the more comprehensive diagnostic mammogram. As Tara had ordered the screening mammogram for me, she had already been called to add a diagnostic mammogram and put a rush on it—a privilege of working at a health institution.

Fortunately, that morning, they had an immediate opening, or maybe they just tried to accommodate me so as not to raise my anxiety even more. Looking back, my worry must have posed a pretty strong contrast to the cheerful and in-charge doctor I normally was and who would come by to discuss someone *else's* mammograms.

The procedure was quick and professional—only a few minutes. The radiology technician, a delightful woman originally from Russia, tried to be as sensitive as possible, knowing that my name was on countless mammograms ordered at this facility. We chatted casually about how patients dreaded mammograms, no matter how gentle the procedure was done—the pain, discomfort, or even humiliation. We both laughed nervously, gallows humor.

After the mammogram, I was asked to wait for the results. I've had to give so much bad news over the years. Doctors are trained in best practices of how to give bad news and I've tried every which way of doing it—being casual, upbeat, giving in to the sadness that I felt, or just saying it matter-of-factly. There are thousands of easy ways to give good news—all ways of giving bad news are uniquely difficult. I loathe giving bad news over the phone and used to ask patients to come in for a discussion; I know now, at least for me, the venue doesn't matter—just do it sooner rather than later.

The radiologist, one of the faculty who was not usually at this location on Mondays, joined me in a small waiting room. She introduced herself as Dr. O'Riordan. We had not met before. *I probably should know my colleagues*, I thought for a moment, but that day everything seemed a blur. All I can remember about what she said was that the mammogram had several areas that "looked a bit unusual." She then suggested we go back and look at the films together. There were areas of microcalcifications, aka microcalcs—tiny calcium deposits—which, on a mammogram, look like white speckles and can be the hallmark of cancer. Looking at the mammograms again, she ordered an ultrasound. She said she could not be sure.

The more intricate, time-consuming MRI wasn't indicated yet because, of course, I still wasn't "high risk." Working like a ship's sonar, ultrasound uses sound waves to detect lumps and lymph nodes that can be missed by a mammogram. Another quick and easy test. As I lay motionless on the examining table, the radiologist used the handheld ultrasound probe to search carefully for any lumps in the breast and high up in the armpit. My focus went back and forth from the images on the screen to the expression on her face. After reviewing the images intensely for several minutes, she said with more reassurance, "No clearly abnormal areas on the ultrasound, and no enlarged lymph nodes in your axilla."

Relief washed over me, because even if I did have cancer, at least it had not spread yet and there were no large tumors.

"But what about that abnormal mammogram?" I asked. "Was it just an error, a false reading?"

"No," she said, looking straight at me, her face somber.

The mammogram was definitely not normal—she still wasn't "too worried"—but "just to be on the safe side"—she wanted to "have another test, a more definitive test." Oh, the language of a practiced physician. Much of the art and science of being a doctor is to recognize the true communication of nonverbal language. I studied her face. And different from her words, I saw a complex mixture of worry, pity, and support in her eyes. She tried in vain to hide it and be reassuring. She was just completing her training in radiology. After so many years in practice, I have long learned very few of us can truly hide concerns. As for me, I will just never be able to pull that off, because I have no "poker face."

Acutely aware of how much each twinge in my doctor's face meant, I also knew very well what "test" she wanted for me—taking a sample of the lesions and looking at them under the microscope. A stereotactic biopsy.

"Can we do it now?" I asked.

She nodded. Instinctively, I crossed my arms in front of my chest before agreeing.

I'd ordered tumor biopsies hundreds of times. It takes only the tapping of a few computer keys and my electronic signature. Easy. Actually having one, as I was learning about many things, is quite different. Depending upon the location, size, number of lumps, medical condition, or the doctor's preference, three primary types of biopsies are possible: *fine-needle aspiration biopsy* (a tiny needle used to draw out a few cells); *core-needle biopsy* (when taking out a cylinder of tissue); or surgical biopsy, better known as a *lumpectomy* or open biopsy (when a tumor is cut out with a scalpel). Mine was to be a core-needle biopsy, or as it turned out, twelve of them.

Wearing an examination gown open at the front, I lay down on the table for the procedure, feeling completely vulnerable. While the radiologist numbed my skin with lidocaine, I glanced over to the instrument tray and to the core gun—a large metal needle with a smaller, bevel-tipped needle inside. The outer needle is four inches long, about the diameter of one of those Starbucks coffee straws, but a dull, metallic gray instead of the familiar green. Each time the inner needle shoots out into the body, it makes a loud *click* or *snap*, like a pellet gun. The thought of this contraption going into my chest made me feel rather queasy.

After making a small incision with a scalpel, the doctor gently inserted the core gun deep into my chest—close to my heart.

I tried not to look. After what seemed an eternity, she told me she'd reached the "area of interest" (aka possible tumor) and pressed a button. *Click*—the biopsy needle shot out and grabbed a piece of tissue from inside me about half an inch long. Its bounty in tow, the needle retracted back into the larger needle, and the core gun was pulled out.

I decided then that the only thing worse than reading a description of a core biopsy, is actually having one.

One down, eleven more to go—yes, that *click* rang out like a gunshot twelve times before I would be done. With each sample, I felt worse. So much was flashing by in my mind, all scenarios far more dramatic than I'd ever imagined before. What if the radiologist pointed it in the wrong direction and shot into my heart? It probably never happens, but what is more likely, what if this sizable needle hit a large blood vessel or damaged a nerve?

How poorly I'd prepared patients all these years before sending them for biopsies, giving them statistics and anatomical terms rather than a statement that there are no two ways around this: "Breast biopsies are not a small thing—they hurt."

Statistically, these biopsies rarely cause significant complications, but they often cause bleeding and bruising. Once again, I tried calming myself with numbers, a professional habit, maybe more a crutch—a 5 percent chance of complication means that 95 patients in 100 will be perfectly fine. And yet, as the person with that core gun being shot into my chest, I was not reassured. I took a deep breath and concentrated on a ceiling tile, then on the glare of the light. I cast my gaze in search of anything to relieve my anxiety. After all, I worked at this hospital and didn't want word getting around that I was a big baby! Being a doctor usually demands being calm and cool-headed even in stressful situations. So why didn't I bring somebody, a friend, or maybe my husband? That could've helped. No, I just marched over here with a mission in mind—thinking of myself as invincible.

Looking back, it wasn't truly painful until the ninth extraction. (And yes, I was counting.) Number nine felt completely different. It actually hurt quite a bit. And by the look of the operator's face after that *click* sounded, she knew it—the needle probably had hit a blood vessel, not uncommon in this procedure going deep into breast tissue. The small incision started to ooze, so she put her fingers on my right breast and pressed down hard to stop the bleeding, casting her gaze away. Again, I became acutely aware of how patients seek reassurance in every twinge in the face of a doctor, even in an invisible face. She let go and quickly got three more cores, after which she continued to press hard on my chest. By no actual fault of hers, she *had* hit a vein, and it took over an hour of pressure before my bleeding stopped. Drastically prolonging my agony. The thought that I could have cancer slowly began to sink in.

Helplessly overcome by fears, I thought about my children. They were still so young. How they would cope; did I raise them to be independent enough? Could they each find their own way? Would my husband manage? How many times was I absentminded or insensitive to their needs? Suddenly, my sense of immortality shattered and I understood the worst of fears and the best of joys. I thought of all the many things left to accomplish before I died. For the first time since that initial phone call, I felt tears welling up in my eyes.

So, there I was, flat on my back on the table alone in my thoughts, with a determined strong woman pressing down on my chest with the three long fingers of her left hand, while using her right hand to write orders so my samples could be processed by the pathologist. In the meantime, my twelve tissue samples were sent for their own X-ray to confirm that the suspicious calcifications were indeed in the specimens taken out of my breast. Tara briefly looked into the room to check on me. Realizing that the radiologist was not yet done, she left again, telling me that she would be waiting for me in the medical hub room.

A few minutes later, the radiology technician confirmed that the biopsies indeed contained the microcalcs the radiologist was trying to capture. Now the tissue needed to be "fixed" (preserved in formalin, a formaldehyde solution), cut into the thin slices, and placed on a glass slide to be looked at under the microscope. Once this had been accomplished, I had to wait for the pathologist to carefully examine all the tissue and determine whether it was cancer and if so, what type, what size, and how aggressive. Usually this would take about a week, often longer. After collecting all the tools and samples, everyone left. The bleeding had finally stopped, and I was ready to leave.

Since I hadn't planned on being there in the first place, I'd made no provisions to cancel my clinic appointments and had patients scheduled all afternoon in the hall next to the radiology suite. It was getting closer to the first appointment at 12:30 pm, and predictably my pager beeped to confirm that my first patient was here. The immediacy of my other life, my life as a physician, returned. Feeling sore and with a bruise about to form, I placed an ice pack under my shirt and walked over to my practice to see my own patients. As I walked over, Tara was standing in our hallway waiting for me. She gave me an encouraging smile. My chest began to hurt and I wondered whether I really could manage a full clinic with patients this afternoon.

Tara's voice broke into my thoughts: "This is going to be okay. No big tumor in the breast, and no mass in your armpit. Do you want to go home?"

Taking a deep breath and straightening my shoulders, I shook my head. "No, I think I can handle this!"

She looked at me; agreeing, with understanding in her eyes: "Okay then, on to business. Let's go; your next patient's ready."

With my most cheerful and upbeat smile, I entered the examining room to my first patient for that day.

Kate was a thirty-eight-year-old-woman with a recent diagnosis of Stage III breast cancer. She had seen a local oncologist and liked him, but she wanted a second opinion from a well-known breast cancer center. Kate's sister was with her, and so all through the visit, two sets of very blue eyes were looking at me apprehensively. The siblings were armed with questions and an inch-thick stack of internet printouts with the latest research on breast cancer.

With an indulgent glance at the stack of paper in front of Kate and a reassuring smile, I leaned back in my chair and looked at both of them: "Would you please tell me what happened so far?

Kate told me that she had noted her skin dimpling about a couple of months back; she was not certain whether she really could tell that she had a lump. Her primary care doctor immediately sent her to a breast surgeon who found a 10 cm (approximately 4-inch) tumor that had spread to two of her lymph nodes. When she told me her story, it wasn't lost on me that the tumor they "found" was almost the same size as her breast. I asked her several questions: how long ago she noted the dimpling, how quickly the lump grew, whether she had any pain, redness, swelling, nipple discharge. Did she have any other medical problems, and pertinent family history? Once I examined her, it was very clear that she had a very large mass in her right breast, palpable nodules in her right armpit (referred to as axilla in the medical report), and a tiny nodule in the area above her collarbone. I explained what I found, choosing my words carefully and looking at both of them. She must have seen the concern in my face.

"I'm willing to do anything," she said anxiously. "No matter how difficult or painful."

Suddenly, there it was again, my confidence. I relaxed my face, and began reassuring this lovely, young mother of two toddlers. I knew she would become a long-term patient; despite my findings, her chances of surviving this breast cancer with a good response to chemotherapy were still high, over 75 percent in ten years. Reassuring myself with statistics and knowledge, I grabbed a pen and paper and began outlining the next steps with them both, three heads huddled together creating a game plan. We talked about the principle and purpose of chemotherapy, the need for reducing her estrogen over the next five to ten years, and whether she should have the mastectomy many of her friends had suggested.

I recommended a course of chemotherapy before surgery to shrink her tumor and assured her that she'd likely be able to continue working, though she could lose her hair. After the chemotherapy and radiation, she'd then take a pill once a day to prevent this cancer, and any future incidents, from ever returning. I then asked Kate what her local doctor had recommended, and she gladly admitted that it was pretty much the same plan. Smiling, I said, "Wonderful, you will be in good hands and you could choose to be treated closer to home."

"I will always be there for backup," I added, seeing the uncertainty in her sister's face.

I learned during my routine history intake that the siblings had no family history of breast cancer, but their father had died in his forties. Since Kate was only in her thirties at the time of her diagnosis, I proposed that we test her for a faulty BRCA gene and called the genetic counselor to talk to her about the test. We completed the consultation, more relaxed and in good spirits. Along the way, I'd even managed to reassure myself about my own situation. I couldn't be worse off than this young woman, and feeling confident she'd do well—then, why shouldn't I as well?

Over the last fifteen years I've had countless discussions on how to treat breast cancer. I've watched women cope with the side effects of therapy, deal with the loss of precious body parts, and struggle because chemotherapy caused early-onset menopause—all side effects of interfering with estrogen levels to starve the tumor of this hormone, which exacerbates its growth. The goal of early-stage breast cancer therapy focuses on eradicating every tumor cell that may have escaped into the rest of the body, to prevent these cells from settling in other organs and metastasizing. It is the spreading of malignant cells that ultimately leads to the death of a patient; and our best chance of preventing these metastases is at the time of the initial diagnosis.

In a very short period of time, Kate and I devised a road map to span the next ten years of treatment, and discussed how to acquire survival strategies and coping mechanisms.

As walked back to the car at the end of a long clinic, I prepared myself for the anguished wait until the results of my biopsy would be in. Driving home that evening, I thought of the fact that my dad's mother actually had had breast cancer. It was just that no one ever talked about it.

Chapter 2

Mastectomy, Still Needed?
Surgical Approaches to Breast Cancer

I was seven years old when my grandmother, my dad's mom, Gertrud, was diagnosed with breast cancer. It was 1971, and she had just turned sixty-five. Grandma lived in Berlin and would usually spend summers with us in Switzerland. The weeks of her visits were a mixed blessing. She always came with a lot of sweets, but her indulging us with expensive chocolates was interspersed with a cool stream of discipline. She did not condone the lax upbringing and informal dress code we enjoyed in Switzerland: I grew up two villages away from Heidi's land, and like her we drank a lot of milk and spent most of our spare time outdoors in the foothills of the Alps, "running wild," according to Grandma.

But when Grandma was around, my parents seemed to remember a lot more rules. Our rooms had to be spotless, our fingernails scrubbed shiny clean; even our dog, a huge Great Dane, seemed to sit mannerly and did not dare to drool. Despite her diminutive size, Grandma was an imposing woman. Even now, when on occasion I think of slipping up with my diet or my office looks disorderly, I see those deep green eyes in her ageless face leveled on me—and I'm reminded that I could do so much better.

Grandma was not unkind; rather, as my mother would say to us over and over again, she "came from a different time." Her husband had died during World War II, leaving her a widow with a small child and no means of her own. Without a complaint, she survived the Hitler years in Berlin; she watched her friends disappear and her own grandmother die from starvation.

The summer of her breast cancer diagnosis was no different. One day during her visit with us, when she was getting dressed, Gertrud felt a tiny, hard lump in her right breast. If she was worried or even panicked, we never knew. Abruptly, she cut her visit short for "a problem that needed attention"—something I'd always somehow remembered despite being a child then. She traveled back to her native Germany to be checked out. And that was it. There was never any talk about it in the family, not even hushed conversations between my parents. As was typical for those days, there was little public discussion of cancer in general. I only learned about her cancer many years later, in an unrelated discussion with my mother about her own health (my mother was the only one Grandma ever told the details to). During those years there were no family rallies for support or neighbors bringing food during therapy, as I see with my patients now.

When she came back a year later, she seemed different. For one thing, I noted that she never wore short-sleeved shirts again. I specifically remember one holiday we all took together to Spain and wondering why she refused to swim with us. Throughout the entire trip, she sat on the balcony of the hotel or took long walks at the beach, always clad in her staple long-sleeved blouses or dresses, while we splashed in the waves. She'd always loved swimming, and it was so hot . . . yet I didn't put two and two together. When I asked whether Grandma was okay, Mom brushed off my questions, saying this was how people of her generation dressed. Except there were many other older women along the shore who were fairly scantily clad, including some I recognized as Germans.

Maybe if I had been older or more perceptive I also would have noticed how thin her hair and her body had become. Her sweet grandmotherly figure and round face disappeared, leaving her eyes a much deeper shade of green. From then on, although it seemed hardly possible, she was even more disciplined, especially when it came to her health: She obsessed about eating regular meals (no extra calories) and took two-hour daily walks starting precisely at 10:00 am (these were much appreciated by our dog, who faithfully stuck her snout into the door of Grandma's room every day at the appointed time and walked with her).

Having watched so many patients go through a breast cancer diagnosis, I now know that the fears, uncertainties, and physical trauma must have been hugely difficult for her to bear in such extreme isolation. For her there was no understanding spouse, supportive parents, or comforting friends showing up on her doorstep with food and hugs and open ears. Now, I can only marvel at how Gertrud dealt with such a diagnosis. Neither my father nor my mother was involved in her care; not for lack of love, but because of the custom of those days, the word *cancer* was rarely uttered. And probably even more devastating, there was little to no discussion of the emotional and psychological tolls of cancer—how to talk to someone with cancer as a doctor or a loved one without saying the wrong words. As I remember from my medical school years in the 1980s, it was a regular practice for doctors to not tell their patients that they even had cancer. The medical community thought it would be too difficult for a patient to handle such a diagnosis.

Because her diagnosis was such a secret at the time, even now and with all of my access to the most advanced medical tools, I cannot definitively retrace the progress of her disease or treatments. Once when her blouse was blown back by the wind—a rare mishap in her impeccable wardrobe—I caught a glimpse of her right armpit and upper arm. They looked dark purple and scarred. Now I recognize that scarring as the severe burns she must have sustained from the type of radiation therapy that was given in those years. There was also the unevenness of her chest and unusual hollowness under her collarbone, which anyone could see under her clothing, especially with her thin frame; this suggested that she had undergone a radical mastectomy—a procedure that removed the breast, the underlying chest muscle, and lots of the lymph nodes in the adjacent armpit; then to make sure the cancer remained contained, a hefty dose of radiation. Now we know that such drastic measures are no longer necessary—I only wish I could have prevented Grandma from having this monstrous surgery.

When I got older and spent more time with Grandma, she would occasionally mention her breast cancer, but she never left room for me to ask about any details. She died in my last year of medical school of pancreatic cancer. All of these images flashed back to me as I was waiting for my biopsy results.

When you're on the receiving end, waiting for the truth about cancer is truly nerve-racking. One of the most important lessons I learned as a doctor was to clearly prepare patients with a timeline for when to expect biopsy results to come back, and it usually takes one to two weeks. Early in my career, I would often tell patients that we would call as soon as the results were in. I never realized that patients literally would sit by the phone for days, not daring to go out, for fear of missing that call.

The Monday after my biopsy, after an entire week of waiting, including an excruciating weekend, I'd had enough. I decided to track down the pathologist who could give me the results of my test.

I walked into the pathology department and, with a brisk, professional air, asked one of the assistants to pull the reports for "Pamela Munster." As she typed in my name, the report came up on the screen.

"Oh, this one is positive, high grade in many places," she commented. "Do you want me to print you a copy?"

"Yes, please," I answered, not yet fully understanding what I had just heard.

As she came back and handed me the printouts, her eyes fell on my name tag, and I watched her face process the connection she'd first missed.

"My God, they didn't call you yet?" She was so crestfallen; I couldn't tell whether I felt worse for myself or her.

"Oh, I sort of knew. I had gotten the prelim already," I lied, referring to what we call a preliminary read, the results put out by a trainee before the diagnosis is finalized by the attending physician. She visibly relaxed.

"I am so sorry for you," she said, trying to smile encouragingly.

"It's fine, thank you," I muttered as I ran to the bathroom, desperately clinging to the pages in my hand.

In the privacy of my stall, I read every word of the summary of the report and then every word of the text. Then I read it again and checked my name. It was my report. And it was very clear:

> High-grade invasive carcinoma in situ (DCIS) in at
> least 5 of the 12 biopsies that were present for review.
> These lesions are malignant. Immediate further surgi-
> cal exploration is recommended.

These were words I had read so many times on reports, and yet reading them now made them feel like a foreign language.

Landing on a piece of the recommendation—*undergo further surgical evaluation*—is when I came out of my haze and my goal-oriented brain snapped back into focus.

"Surgical exploration" meant I needed a breast surgeon. So I immediately walked down to the clinic to find Tara, who on Monday mornings would be in her office preparing my clinic. She turned around and stared at my teary eyes. Before she even finished reading the entire report, my ever-so-polite nurse practitioner uttered a long string of unceremonious curses. Had I not been so upset, I would have been laughing. She took the report and grabbed my hand and walked me over to the office of our head surgery nurse, Debbie, and showed her the results.

Here my expertise and employment at the institution gave me an edge in many ways. Unlike most patients, I did not need much explanation about what needed to happen next. We briefly discussed which surgeon I wanted to see. Without further delay, Debbie picked up the phone and made several calls to schedule all the appointments I needed to get this taken care of as quickly as possible. But most helpful of all, she let me cry in her arms—and relinquish my role as the doctor to let myself become a patient.

I chose a surgeon with whom I had worked when he was a trainee, who—now at our current institution—was a respected colleague, Dr. Michael Alvarado. I had seen with my own eyes that he had skilled surgical hands and a wonderful bedside manner. Most of all, I liked him as a person, and I fully trusted he would treat me according to the current best medical knowledge while respecting my own wishes.

He called me back and said he would see me the next day, after he had a chance to review all my scans and discuss the findings with the radiologist. I made an appointment and, with Debbie at my side, saw Dr. Alvarado as a patient—no longer as a colleague and former mentor. He asked me many questions: how I felt; whether there was cancer in the family; whether I had previous biopsies; and most important, whether I had noticed any changes in my breast.

"I assume you did not find any lumps, nipple discharge, redness?" he said, referring to the fact that my cancer was detected on a screening mammogram. It is often a lump that brings the patient to the office, but not for me. He examined me for lumps and lymph nodes under my armpits and above my clavicle; I was glad that he couldn't find any, either, and I let go of feeling guilty that I'd missed something myself. Finally, he reviewed all mammogram and ultrasound results with me.

Sitting there in a hospital gown, I listened to my colleague lay out a treatment plan I'd delivered so many times myself. In reviewing what he felt were my best surgical options, Dr. Alvarado told me that he did not think he could do a lumpectomy; it would be much better for me to have a mastectomy. I knew why he recommended this as a doctor, but as the patient sitting in front of him, I asked him to walk me through the options.

As was the case during the time of the radical mastectomy, the kind Grandma had, the goal of today's breast surgery is still to remove all of the tumor. But unlike forty years ago, we now know that there is no need to remove the whole breast or the muscles underneath. Only the abnormal areas have to be removed, and those should be excised completely with no abnormal tissue left behind.

Many eminent breast surgeons battled for years over how much healthy tissue has to be removed to keep the patient cancer free. Dr. William Halsted initially pioneered the radical mastectomy almost two centuries ago. At that time, he and others were convinced that all breast cancers spread from the breast to the lymph nodes and then on to other organs—hence aggressive surgery that removed all of the breast, the underlying muscles, and all the surrounding lymph nodes to prevent the tumors from spreading. Dr. Bernard Fisher and his colleagues argued that breast cancer could also spread to other organs directly through the blood system with or without passing through the lymph nodes, so just doing more surgery in a tumor that had already spread would really not impact the survival of the patient. In a revolutionary act, Dr. Fisher and a large team of colleagues studied hundreds of women in the National Surgical Adjuvant Breast Project. The group successfully showed two things: that the extent of the surgery did not make a difference, and those patients with high-risk cancer needed chemotherapy regardless whether they had a lumpectomy or mastectomy. Thankfully, today no woman needs the dreadful surgery that my grandmother had.

For any woman diagnosed with breast cancer today, there are two options to remove the tumor: a lumpectomy (-*ectomy* means "removing"), or a *mastectomy* (*mastos*- means "breast").

For a lumpectomy, the surgeon typically makes a small incision and then cuts out the tumor. To ensure that the entire tumor is taken out, he hands the piece of tissue that contains the suspicious area to a nurse who then will proceed to "ink the tumor." All six edges of the cancerous lump are dipped in a special color ink. A pathologist then verifies that the lump is a tumor, what type it is, how aggressive, and that there are no cancerous cells at the edge of the lump, called the margin. A *clear, negative,* or *clean margin* means that there are no tumor cells in the inked margins. A *positive margin* means that cancer cells come all the way to the edge of the excised lump and have ink on them. In most cases the pathologist actually specifies how close the tumor comes to the edge in millimeters, such as a 2 mm margin. If the pathology report reads that tumor cells are within in the inked *lateral margin*, this would mean that the tumor comes all the way out to the outside edge. If a positive margin is found, the color of the ink will tell the surgeon where to go back and cut out more tissue.

When part of a tumor is left behind in a margin, it may grow back at that site. A tumor recurrence is twice as likely if there is tumor on the inked margins, so having clear margins is really important. As many as 25 percent of women will have to go back to the operating room and have a positive margin reexcised. Typically, the surgeon then takes the patient back in the next couple of weeks and cuts an extra slice of tissue from the outside part of the cavity. This procedure must be repeated until all margins are clear.

Although every woman should have the option for a lumpectomy—aptly referred to as breast conservation treatment—there are strong medical and nonmedical reasons for a full mastectomy, or complete removal of one or both breasts. In the majority of patients, only one abnormal area is found on the mammogram. Since only this area has to be removed, the choice of surgery is mainly guided by the cosmetic outcome. Ideally, a small tumor is excised with clear margins and the woman still has lots of breast tissue left; taking out the lump does not leave a visible hole or distort the fullness or shape of the breast. If the tumor is sizable and the breast is small, it may be challenging to preserve a good contour. Even in women with larger breasts, if a tumor is very large there may not be much breast tissue left, and the patient could be left with a big hollow cavity and a noticeable difference in size and shape. Fortunately, nowadays with newer surgical techniques, plastic surgeons can rearrange the tissue to make sure that the shape and size of the breast remains intact, or if the woman has any excessive fat tissue available elsewhere in the body, a trained plastic surgeon will remove the fat from the belly or thigh and use it to fill the hole with a procedure called fat grafting.

More commonly now, if a tumor is so big that removing it would leave too little breast tissue behind, the oncologist will often suggest treating the patient with chemotherapy for three to six months before surgery to shrink the tumor with what is called neoadjuvant chemotherapy. Neoadjuvant chemotherapy is highly effective in killing tumor cells and thereby making the tumor resectable—meaning its removal would allow breast conservation in many more patients.

A key factor to not overlook in the flurry of decision-making is that the choice of surgery often will not affect the survival rates. Women should not choose to have a mastectomy because they think it may increase their chance of survival. There is extensive research showing that most women who have a mastectomy will not live longer statistically that those who choose a lumpectomy. If a tumor is totally removed and the patient has four to six weeks of radiation on that breast, the survival rate will be the same as if she had a mastectomy in most cases.

Lumpectomy, despite requiring radiation, overall has fewer complications, causes less emotional distress, and is much more cost effective than a mastectomy. Another layer of complication with mastectomy is that it typically requires another surgery for reconstruction; the procedure itself also carries a more than twofold risk of complication than lumpectomy.

However, there are truly patients for whom a lumpectomy is not possible. Dr. Alvarado told me that he could not do a lumpectomy in my case: "Actually, I probably could do a lumpectomy on you—I'd just have to do five or six lumpectomies to cut out all the areas that are abnormal. If I have to cut out five areas of at least half an inch, you may not be left with much," he said with a sheepish grin.

I stared at him with in utter disbelief at this feeble attempt of humor, and it took me a moment to realize what he meant. What are friends for, right? However, his gentle jest broke my tension; so, I muttered something I would not want to repeat and snapped back to reality.

I realized my mind had wandered off trying to grapple with the fact of what was actually happening to me. Before my eyes was a scroll of visions ranging from being surgically mutilated, hearing my own eulogy, and seeing my husband and kids trying to adjust to a new life. Instead I forced myself to pay attention to the person who was trying to help prevent all that from becoming reality.

Sensing that I was rapidly losing focus, the surgeon started to explain in more concrete detail why I could not have a lumpectomy, wisely appealing to my logical mind.

"Your mammogram suggested that you have at least five areas that appeared abnormal," he said more slowly. "I am afraid, as you know, that regardless of whether this is actually invasive cancer or just DCIS, the goals of surgery remain the same. We want to remove all the abnormal areas before they transform into more aggressive tumors and spread to other organs. Unfortunately, in your case, removing all the abnormal tissue would be surgically very challenging and cause enough disfiguration that cosmetically, you would be better served with a mastectomy and reconstruction."

Dr. Alvarado was hopeful that as in the biopsy, he would find only DCIS —ductal carcinoma in situ, what we consider Stage 0 or noninvasive cancer—during the final surgery. Belying that hopeful tone, however, were the justified concerns that with five abnormal areas seen on the mammogram, I was at a fairly high risk of his finding more tumors in other places during surgery itself and of having even more aggressive tumors.

So I asked him directly, "Assume for a moment that I am not a colleague, please, and walk me through the scenario of what would happen if I did nothing and just waited a while."

I already knew that I really did not have a choice. He did not need to say it, but I needed to hear the facts spoken aloud to wrap my head around giving up my breast. Recommending a mastectomy to someone else and having one are really two entirely different things.

"There are mainly two issues," he began. "While it looks from the biopsies and mammogram that all your lesions may be Stage Zero, only after we take them out can the pathologist tell us for certain whether or not all of these lesions are tumors. And second, from the initial biopsy, it looks like several of your tumors are at least high-grade DCIS, and if not already invasive, the chance is high that they will turn invasive. With five lesions already visible on mammogram, the chance of having more tumors in the near future is very high—probably around thirty percent in the next five years. So, for you the question really is not surgery or not—but rather, *what* surgery. And I am afraid that with one of your lesions being so far back on the muscle, a lumpectomy would technically very challenging." He also reminded me of the higher recurrence rate if the margins were positive.

And then he paused, silently giving me time to grasp the meaning of what he was saying.

So sometimes a lumpectomy is simply not possible, and a mastectomy is medically necessary—as in my case with *multifocal* (meaning more than one tumor in the same quadrant of the breast) and *multicentric* disease (multiple tumors throughout the breast). It will then not really matter if these are high-grade or low-grade tumors, aggressive or invasive—they just need to come out.

Although I'd said nothing in reply, he continued, "If you decide on mastectomy, the most important next step will be to talk to the plastic surgeon and discuss what options you have for reconstruction. And in your case, given how many abnormal areas you have in this breast, an MRI of the other breast may be a good idea to make sure that nothing was missed on the mammogram."

I left his office with very mixed emotions and a referral to see a plastic surgeon to discuss reconstruction. The good news was that I really did not have invasive cancer—at least as far as we knew. Nonetheless, I was facing the surgical removal of at least one breast and maybe both.

When counseling patients in the past about what to do with the other breast, I would always impress on them to consider all the options, yet I always secretly thought that I would choose a double mastectomy if it were me. But now it was me, and I walked out forcing myself to start thinking on what I really wanted.

Admittedly, at first glance my quick decision may seem like an emotional overreaction. And it is not easy, even medically, to justify how my Stage 0 cancer turned into a double mastectomy; just compare it to Kate, who despite having highly aggressive Stage III cancer needed only a lumpectomy. But I actually had some of my reasoning skills intact, and there's good reason to do more surgery for a lower-stage breast cancer.

About 6 percent of the 250,000 women in the US diagnosed with breast cancer each year present with tumors that have spread already to other organs (making it Stage IV, or metastatic disease). In these cases, removing the tumor from the breast will not impact survival. It would be like rushing to close the barn after the horses have run off. All patients with Stage IV disease will need treatment for the entire body, not just the breast.

As a breast cancer patient, I was extremely lucky. I was diagnosed with the earliest form of breast cancer and had the option to never have to deal with it again. What reasons for keeping my breasts would override the chance of ultimate peace of mind now? If I waited with surgery, I would need intense screening with MRIs and mammograms, and possibly repeated biopsies, every six months. Why would I want to endure that agony?

The most successful way to treat and prevent breast cancer is finding it early and taking care of it before the tumor spreads to other organs. Breast cancer is curable as long as it stays in the breast or at least does not go beyond the lymph nodes in the armpit on the same side of the body. If all of the tumor can be cut out with clear margins and has not spread, then the patient is cured. So, while it seems paradoxical, Kate might have to wait five to ten years until she can stop worrying whether her Stage III invasive cancer may spread and turn into metastatic cancer, whereas my Stage 0 cancer, once removed, almost certainly would never come back or turn into metastatic disease.

Prior to Stage IV, though, surgical interventions are possible and more likely to be curable. Stage I is any tumor less than 2 cm without spread to any lymph nodes. Stage II is a tumor that measures between 2 and 5 cm and may have spread to the lymph nodes in the axilla. Stage III is a tumor more than 5 cm or many lymph nodes with tumors. While our goal still is to remove all the tumors, with increasing size and number of lymph nodes there is a higher likelihood that tumor cells escape and settle in other organs and become metastatic. The size of the tumor and the number of lymph nodes involved then will guide the need and choice of chemotherapy. The risk of dying from breast cancer is greatly increased with increasing tumor size, from around 10 percent in ten years for Stage I to greater than 30 percent for Stage III. Over the last few years, newer technologies have discovered that the patterns of genes and proteins in breast cancer can also tell whether a tumor is aggressive. We now know that a low-risk gene expression pattern in a big tumor carries a better prognosis, whereas a Stage I tumor with an aggressive pattern may need special attention despite its being small.

I was among the roughly sixty thousand women per year in the US who are fortunate to have found their cancer at a stage when it is still in a contained, ductal carcinoma in situ (DCIS) or Stage 0 disease. *Ductal carcinoma in situ* means the cells that line the milk ducts of the breast have become cancerous, but they have not invaded the surrounding breast tissue.

While for invasive cancer, lumpectomy and radiation has a comparable survival than mastectomy, this is because nearly all women get hormonal therapy and maybe chemotherapy. For DCIS, a mastectomy is sufficient and does not require hormonal therapy; a woman with DCIS treated with a lumpectomy should also get radiation therapy to the same breast and then five years of hormonal therapy, such as tamoxifen, an antiestrogen with the goal to reduce estrogen in the body.

It does seem like a lot to go through for any women with Stage 0 disease. If it is not yet cancer, why so much therapy? And what would happen if a woman just could not do it and decided to do nothing?

There is increasing debate whether DCIS could be left untreated, though not much data exist on this option, as very few surgeons would really feel comfortable doing nothing for these patients. Still, there are rare circumstances in which we know it is not wrong to forgo surgery entirely. DCIS itself comes in three categories: *high grade, intermediate grade*, and *low grade*. Surgery may be omitted if the DCIS is truly low grade, as very large studies recently have shown, but that only occurs in one in five women. A study that took place between 1988 and 2011 observed a group of fifty-seven thousand women with DCIS, wherein all but 2 percent did not have surgery. Comparing that group to those who underwent either a mastectomy or lumpectomy, for all but the women with low-risk DCIS, those undergoing the surgery fared much better. At ten years, 7 percent of those without surgery died of breast cancer, whereas less than 1 percent of those undergoing surgery died. Looking more closely at who had surgery, it appeared that the death rate among those with high-grade tumors who did not have surgery was even higher, saving about 8 in 100 patients from breast cancer deaths in ten years. By contrast, patients with low-risk tumors could actually forgo surgery without taking extra risks, and the chance of dying from breast cancer with low-risk DCIS was about 1 to 2 percent regardless of surgery. Many studies are underway to search for factors other than size and grade that may dictate the need for surgery.

This study answered my question of what would happen if I chose to do nothing, no surgery at all. With high-risk DCIS at multiple sites, I would have a nearly 10 percent chance of dying from breast cancer before I turned sixty and a more than 30 percent chance that any of these lesions turned into an aggressive tumor. And if I were diagnosed with invasive cancer, I would likely end up with chemotherapy and for sure would require five to ten years of tamoxifen in addition to the mastectomy.

There is an infamously long list of much-feared side effects in the package insert of tamoxifen, and many have been experienced by patients: weight gain, moodiness, depression, hot flashes, among others. Hearing stories of friends and relatives treated with tamoxifen, many of my patients have expressed strong objections to using it for the prevention of breast cancer; they would rather consider extensive surgery and losing the breast.

My combination of circumstances was unusual; I did not have the option of breast conservation. Medically, I would need a mastectomy because I had several areas of tumors.

However for any woman with a small tumor that can easily be removed, a mastectomy should not be needed. So why are so many mastectomies still being done? Over the last ten years, there has actually been a considerable increase in the number of mastectomies that are performed in the US—and particularly striking is the increase in the rate of double mastectomies. This begs of course the question, who is driving this decision: doctor or patient?

My decision would be to have a one-sided or a bilateral (two-sided) mastectomy—one that has troubled many women and doctors and has been much under public debate. From patient surveys and registry studies, we know that the reasons are multifold. There are several factors steering a woman toward a bilateral mastectomy. The most commonly stated reason by almost all women is having peace of mind. Unfortunately, the same surveys also showed that many women actually erroneously think that a bilateral mastectomy will prolong their lives. It is imperative for both the surgeon and the patient to discuss whether a bilateral mastectomy in the individual patient would impact her dying from breast cancer. However, peace of mind can entail not needing further biopsies or mammograms. A bilateral mastectomy for DCIS may mean no tamoxifen. Women with a family history tend to worry more. Other factors included cosmetic reasons, a younger age, and having larger breasts—more women in these groups all tended to have bilateral mastectomies.

Now having been on both sides of the fence, as a doctor and patient, I can point to several reasons why a woman would choose a double mastectomy, even those I hadn't implicitly known from patients. As an oncologist who sees patients for many years after their surgery, I have absolutely no doubt that two reconstructed breasts after bilateral mastectomies are cosmetically more similar, hence the surgery at first glance is less apparent when the patient is fully clothed. Only with very extensive surgery on the contralateral side can most women look symmetrical with a one-sided reconstruction. When one breast has a different shape and is in a different position, asymmetry is much more difficult to hide. It's hard not to feel self-conscious in a cocktail dress or tank top, and unthinkable for me not to feel so in a yoga top. Creating evenness both in large-breasted or in thin, small-breasted women can be challenging. Mastectomies are much larger procedures, and two or three surgeries are needed for a full reconstruction including a lift or even a cosmetic implant.

For many of my patients, including myself, peace of mind is an important factor even if a woman is very clear that the bilateral mastectomy will not necessarily impact survival. There is the continued need for ongoing screening for someone who had a lumpectomy or no surgery on the other side. For me after having just gone through mammograms, ultrasounds, MRIs, and twelve core biopsies, the thought of more such screening every six to twelve months in the future was really hard to accept.

And lastly, the decision comes at the time when many women are really vulnerable. All the reassurance in the world that the risk for breast cancer in other breast is really low is hardly convincing to someone who has been just diagnosed with breast cancer. Like me, most women probably did not expect this to happen to either of her breasts. So taken all together, it is not surprising that so many women choose a mastectomy during a time when they feel most vulnerable and scared. At this moment I was confident that a mastectomy would be the end of my cancer story: no further mammograms, no ultrasounds, no need for radiation therapy, and no tamoxifen. If I had a bilateral mastectomy, I would not have to worry about breast cancer ever again. For me, there was no question that giving up my breasts would result in peace of mind.

But I still paused, as I would ask every woman in my situation to do, to ask myself: Would I still feel this way in the months and years down the line? There is no going back after mastectomy, and what if in five years research brings other treatments making a mastectomy obsolete? What if I made a decision just a few years, or months, or weeks before a new discovery came along and let me keep my breasts?

As I left Dr. Alvarado's office sure of my surgical decision, I considered how often patients had asked me what I would do in their shoes. Normally, I could only reply, "It is hard to tell; I am not in your shoes." But now I was in exactly those shoes. I had the benefit of having seen firsthand the consequences from a one-sided mastectomy and those from a double mastectomy, the impact this procedure has on a woman in the years immediately after surgery and then in the long term. What appears important early on may not remain important as the time goes by.

I still don't make suggestions on what a patient should choose, but I more thoroughly present the details of what each choice entails, discuss the benefits and limitations, share my experience, and try to find out what is important for the person sitting in front of me. Here I would implore every patient to complete all the visits with the surgery teams, see the plastic surgeon to discuss all options, but then take some time to make sure that the decision to do extra surgery is right for now and will still hold in years to come.

What I hope to impart is the notion that the type of surgery should be a very personal choice, tailored to individual needs and guided by medical circumstances for every patient and with the guidance, not dictation, of her doctor. And most important, the final decision should be made from a truly informed choice rather than misconception of false benefits of the procedure.

And so I went and began to discuss the options for reconstructions with the plastic surgeon—and in addition, do what I always do in the face of difficult decisions: to try to step away for a bit to find distance and time to reflect.

Chapter 3

Reconstruction:
Surgical Options and Decisions

B arely a week had passed since I first learned about my breast cancer, and despite my clear-headedness about my decision to permanently rid myself of cancer, I had to force myself to take a step and think about all the options in detail—the precautions I'd advise a patient to take.

Heeding my own advice, I needed to hear about my options for reconstructions.

First, I needed to find the right plastic surgeon for me—someone who would work well with my breast surgeon, but also someone I could level with on my own terms. As I called Dr. Alvarado to ask for a recommendation, I remembered having a discussion with one of my young patients about choosing a plastic surgeon for her breast reconstruction. I had told her that choosing a good plastic surgeon was a bit like choosing a good school for your kids: There is so much more to the decision than the quantitative value of the school's reputation and teachers. What matters just as much is the quality of the environment: the other kids, the other moms, the school board. Finding the right fit can be incredibly overwhelming, which is why in the end, even after doing our homework, most of us rely on the recommendations of a trusted friend or professional or go walk into the school and get a feel for it.

Finding the right plastic surgeon is equally complex. He or she should be able and willing to perform all the possible surgeries that could be an option, or refer you to a colleague if he or she does not perform this kind of surgery. The plastic surgeon should be able to operate and work well with your breast surgeon (often called the "dream team"). And most of all, you should be comfortable with your plastic surgeon so as to be able to discuss your wishes and express concerns and worries, now and later. In the end, both the patient and plastic surgeon will be happiest if the surgery is technically ideal for the patient's anatomy and at the same time fulfills the patient's needs and lifestyle. However, getting there can sometimes be rocky, as during this time of decision-making, most women are still stunned from their diagnosis and filled with a sense of urgency. Often patients want this surgery to happen as soon as possible, even if it leaves less time than is truly needed to weigh their options and permanent consequences. This is the time to have a long view.

I was privileged as a patient to have my insider view; on the other hand, I had to put myself into the hands of a colleague. While there were many advantages of being treated at my medical center, the disadvantage was that everybody knew me. For a long while, I had debated whether I should go to another institution, but the added challenges of having surgery at a different place made life just too complicated.

So, I did what the breast care team recommended to everybody else: "Talk to your breast surgeon." I implicitly trusted mine to recommend the "right" plastic surgeon for me.

When Dr. Alvarado called me back, he sounded a bit apprehensive but genuinely relieved to hear from me. I explained I had pretty much made up my mind to proceed with the mastectomy on my breast with the ductal carcinoma in situ (DCIS) but wanted to have a better understanding of my options for the side without cancer.

"We have a new plastic surgeon working in our other office who just arrived a couple of weeks ago from the East Coast, and he's great to work with. Let's talk with him about this," he advised.

"Ah, yes, I heard he is coming and saw his name on our roster. Did he actually start?"

"Yes, but he wouldn't have had reason to meet you. He mainly sees patients on our other campus. You also may feel more comfortable with someone you don't work with every day. Hani is a very competent surgeon, and he can *stand* his ground! Even when his patient is a doctor, too."

I picked up on Dr. Alvarado's implication that I could be a bit . . . overbearing. I had to grin; I do have opinions on most things. He was used to seeing me in charge of a large research team or as a consultant for mutual patients. He couldn't know just how overwhelmed I was with all this. It took a little time for both of us to accept that this was not another consultation about a mutual patient—this was me, and I was his patient now to take care of.

From observing patients over years, I knew that trust is an important element in the relationship between a patient and doctor. From a doctor's perspective, I naturally feel closer to patients who trust me. Any patients who cannot trust their doctor should think of finding a different one. Now that I was the patient, I slowly began to transfer the responsibility for my care to my fellow professionals, and once done, I could more easily accept the guidance and support I really needed—even for someone who knew all the options and possibilities. I'd made up my mind to have a bilateral mastectomy. Yet not for the first time, I was still desperately hoping that this was all just a bad dream and soon I would wake up, shaken and sweaty, but with my old life back.

Hanging up with Dr. Alvarado, I immediately called the office of Dr. Hani Sbitany and asked for an appointment. When he called me back shortly after saying he'd just had a cancellation and he could see me today, I jumped at the opening. Waiting was just not my thing.

A few hours later, I was sitting in our examination room, shivering in a gown, my palms clammy. I was trying hard to keep cool, making jokes with our medical assistants who clearly worked just as hard to hide how sorry they felt for me. I wasn't their physician anymore, but one of "them"—the patients.

A brisk knock announced Dr. Sbitany, who came into the room with a nurse from the plastic surgery department, Janet, who I knew quite well. The surgeon was tall and had a reassuring smile. We chatted a bit about his transfer from his prior institution, ignoring the fact that I was his potential patient and not just a fellow doctor he was meeting for the first time. I wondered what he had been told about me. An older colleague, a well-established professor, a breast cancer expert, an opinionated/difficult woman . . . ? Or just someone else with cancer?

"It is nice to finally meet you," he said. "I am sorry it is under these circumstances."

"Yes, me too, but I am glad you could fit me in so quickly. If my husband can call you later, this would be great."

He told me that he had shared cases with my husband, who is also an oncologist and was in Dr. Sbitany's department. He promised that he would call him later and give him a summary of the plan.

"Michael told me that he would need to do a mastectomy on the right side, and that you were leaning toward a bilateral mastectomy." Dr. Sbitany glanced at me for confirmation.

I reminded myself that I came here not quite leaning toward anything, but open to suggestions.

"Would you please outline the options for me?" I interrupted him. "I have my thoughts of what I want, but would like to hear your opinion."

Assessing me for a moment, he said, "The choice is between silicone implants or a transfer of your own fat tissue to rebuild the breast. You may be a bit thin for any natural flaps or fat transfer, I'm afraid, so implants may be a better choice for you."

"Oh, and here I thought one is never too thin," I said to break through the tension of so frank an evaluation of my body.

Janet laughed out loud and grinned at me.

"Actually, quite true in this case and not just flattery," Dr. Sbitany retorted with a smile, trying to put me more at ease.

Nonetheless, I felt even more exposed.

Although I had treated patients with breast cancer and examined many others for years, I was not quite prepared for how vulnerable I would feel having this doctor's professional eyes on me. I was also not yet aware that it would take me months to get used to this. At that moment, all I really wanted was to just hide under a blanket and not deal with any of it.

Wishing I had brought a friend, I looked at Janet for support and asked Dr. Sbitany, "Assuming for a moment that not all the options are feasible for me, would you please describe the options that you think would work best for me?" Seeing my rising distress, he looked at me for a long moment and gently asked, "May I examine you?"

I nodded, and he and Janet stepped out to give me privacy while I changed.

At the sight of the hospital gown, I started to feel uneasy. I'd worn them before when I'd had my children, and talked with gowned women every day most of my life. But this felt different. Each pregnancy left me with a gorgeous child. Usually I would be on the doctor's side of the examining table when it came time to conduct a breast exam, which was sensitive for so many reasons. This time I was sitting on the examining table, for the first time frightfully aware how much of my womanhood was at stake here. I have never given that much thought of what defined me as a female. I had always just comfortably been one. Now about to lose my breasts, I thought about how I would feel afterward. Is that why this was so hard?

Suddenly, there was a knock on the door. I quickly wrapped myself in the blue and white hospital gown.

After the exam, I sat on the table and listened as Dr. Sbitany explained his opinions.

As requested, he outlined the principles of each procedure for me.

The goal of any mastectomy and reconstruction is to completely remove all breast tissue, cancerous or not, and then rebuild a breast. But over the last few years, more and more women have chosen less drastic procedures that minimize the removal of skin, which reduce scarring and usually provide a better cosmetic outcome for the reconstructed breast.

In a skin-sparing mastectomy, the nipples and area around the nipple are removed; in a skin- and nipple-sparing mastectomy, they are left intact, though. To lessen the impact of the mastectomy, sparing the skin and nipples has been an important step forward. Yet, nipple-sparing mastectomies are done less frequently. Although these surgeries were described more than fifty years ago, the technique is controversial and many surgeons remain cautious about leaving the nipple, out of fear of the tumor coming back in the nipple. Nipple-sparing mastectomies are not recommended in larger tumors or if the tumor is close to the nipple, for fear of leaving tumor cells behind and later recurrence, but recent studies have shown that the risk of tumors coming back in the nipple after a nipple-sparing mastectomy are fairly low and hopefully more women will be able to save their nipples, and as much skin as possible with minimized risk.

However, there are a few other risks involved in nipple-sparing mastectomies: A major one is the risk that the nipple, or part of it, does not survive all the manipulations during the surgery. Nipple necrosis and loss happens in 5 to 10 percent of patients.

In some women, it is technically difficult to rebuild the breast and have the nipples in the right spot after reconstruction. Sometimes it takes one more surgery to get it right. For those who cannot keep their nipples, rebuilding them is, surgically speaking, fairly easy, and it can be done at any time in the office. Nipples can also be tattooed onto the skin. There are amazing tattoo artists who can create a 3-D appearance of a nipple; on several of my patients, I did a double take before realizing their tattooed nipples weren't real.

Unfortunately, regardless of what type of surgery is performed or the type of reconstruction that is chosen, in most women, the sensation in the nipple is lost completely or partially after a mastectomy. The loss of nipple sensation is for many women the one long-lasting effect that is difficult to deal with. Nipple and breast skin recovery occurs in some patients, but if it happens, it may take years.

The materials used to rebuild the breast includes a saline or silicone implant, or a patient's own fat or muscle transferred from other places, such as the back, belly, or thighs. To rebuild a breast, there is often not enough extra fat to be found. One might think that simply gaining weight just to have enough fat to build a breast from would work as a solution; however, it does not, since the breast will disappear if the woman loses the fat again. And you'd need twice as much fat for bilateral mastectomies. *This does not seem to be the procedure for me*, I thought, my attention fading.

Moreover, fat- and muscle-type reconstructions need open blood vessels for the tissue to survive. In a complicated procedure, whole sections of fat from the belly are transferred to the breast, and the blood vessels in the abdomen are severed and then reattached in the chest. In the increasingly popular reconstruction called a deep inferior epigastric perforator (DIEP) flap, the abdominal fat tissue is transferred without affecting the abdominal muscles; if done well, the surgery leaves the patient with nothing artificial inside her body and very natural-feeling breasts.

To connect the tiniest blood vessels in the fat tissue, much of this surgery is done with a microscope in the operating room—so, needless to say, the procedure requires a specially trained surgeon with expertise in microvascular surgery. Given their intricacy, these surgeries are long, often more than twelve hours, and need monitoring for days after (usually in the ICU) to make sure that the flap survives and the vessels stay open. There are other drawbacks as well. The fat transfer requires a sizable incision in the lower abdomen and leaves a noticeable scar. While the procedure does come with a bonus tummy tuck, healing for the incision takes longer. This procedure can only be done once, so a patient should carefully consider whether she will need more surgery on the other breast at a later time. Furthermore, sometimes the fat tissue dies, leaving uneven areas that need to be refilled by additional surgeries. Women with prior abdominal surgeries are not ideal candidates for this surgery. For those who cannot use their own tissue to rebuild their breasts, silicone implants are now most frequently used.

Still shivering, I pulled my gown closed and interrupted Dr. Sbitany: "If I wanted a fat transfer surgery, would I really be a candidate?"

He looked at me one more time and asked, "Have you and Dr. Alvarado made a decision on what to do on the other side? Is a one-sided mastectomy an option?" I nodded and said that I wanted to know what my options for reconstruction were before finalizing my decisions.

"I may be able to do a one-sided DIEP, but not for a bilateral mastectomy," he replied.

"If I wanted to keep my healthy breast for now, I could not go back later and do another DIEP procedure?" I asked, confirming what I thought I heard him say before.

"Not a DIEP, that is correct. But we could do a latissimus dorsi flap, taking muscle from your back, or we could insert an implant on the other side, if you ever needed to remove the other breast," he added gently.

"If I did the DIEP on the right side and kept my natural left breast, wouldn't I look uneven?"

I pointed out that symmetry was a huge problem for many of my patients in the long run, as having a different size and shape in the breasts is actually quite noticeable.

"Given that I am no longer seventeen, what would it take to make me even?" I mumbled under my breath, pointing out that I was quite aware of the challenges of matching the reconstructed breast to the natural breast.

He nodded, hiding a grin, and then outlined the steps I would need to do on the left side to match the reconstruction of my right breast. Essentially, that would involve a procedure to lift up and tighten the breast tissue, maybe an implant on the left side, some tweaking here and then some there. Surely he did not use the words "tweaking here and there," but at that moment I had visions of a meticulous artist with a knife working to create perfect symmetry. And from talking to patients over the years, I knew I was not that far off.

Over the past few years, more and more women have decided to undergo a mastectomy on the healthy breast as well, just for that reason: to avoid having all those procedures to make the other side maybe comparable. I was listening to all the things I would need to do on my healthy breast just to look symmetrical, while knowing that I would then still need to stay vigilant and have more MRIs and mammograms—and possibly more biopsies. Very quickly, I decided that I did not want more surgeries than absolutely necessary; and I really was looking forward to the time when this would all be over.

Fortunately, I did not object to having implants, and so the complexity of a DIEP procedure did not seem like a good option for me. I worried about having a very long surgery, and how my spending extra days in the hospital would put considerable extra stress on my young daughter. I knew from the past that my skin heals with scars, too, so the idea of a big incision across my belly was not very appealing.

"Okay, I think I get the picture. What would *you* think best for me?" I looked first at Dr. Sbitany and then at Janet. But before they could respond, I added, "I am very strongly leaning toward a bilateral mastectomy. For me, symmetry is really important. Also, I like sports and hope for few restrictions and a short recovery time."

Exercise has always been an important part of my life—for the joy of it and a way to manage stress and anxiety. In my youth, school counselors and psychologists, as well as my mother, made sure I had enough activity and spent as much time as possible outdoors. Growing up in the Alps, this was easy. As long as I can remember, I was on the ski team. Wednesday and Saturday afternoons, I was on the slopes racing through the slalom courses, usually competing on Sundays. When the snow melted and the weather got warmer, I signed up for track and field. I recall a stint of ballet at some point, but my French dance teacher impressed on my parents that this refined activity was not the most ideal for my exuberant temperament.

I still love all sorts of sports and I could not imagine not being able to ski or mountain bike—or showing up to a yoga studio with a lopsided chest.

"With this in mind, then, what do you think would work best for me?"

Janet looked at my chest and then at my face, meeting my gaze. She gave me a faint smile. And for the first time, I became aware of what would become so familiar to me, understanding and empathy in her eyes.

"To be totally honest, I think implants are really the best options for you," said Dr. Sbitany emphatically. "Implants look great on thin people and we will have a lot of choices with size and shapes. You should be able to keep most of your skin and both nipples. I don't think I will need to move the nipples at all. During the time of the mastectomy, we will place an expander under your pec muscles that we slowly inflate—and over the course of three to four months, they will stretch the muscle and skin so we can place the final implant."

"So I will still need another surgery in three months?" I interrupted.

He nodded, explaining that for me a two-stage procedure after a mastectomy would be preferable. The skin and muscle needed to adjust to make enough space for the implant. Also, because the skin would be very thin after the surgery, letting it heal would cause less damage and also limit the chance of nipple necrosis.

Week by week over those three months he would slowly fill the expander with fluid injected through a needle until I reached a volume that I thought would look and feel good on me and what I ultimately would want the final silicone implant to be.

There has been much progress in the development of silicone implants, namely after their having been banned for some time in the '90s for fear of causing "bad reactions" from leaking. After almost two decades of meticulous reporting of all immediate and late side effects, implants are now deemed safe. Blissfully, the less attractive saline implants are now a thing of the past.

Silicone implants usually last about ten years, and at that point, there is an option to exchange them. The newer implants rarely leak and should not cause undue tissue reactions. Many of my patients had silicone implants for way longer than ten years and never really got around to changing them or needed to change them.

Just as I was about to ask about the downside of silicone implants, Dr. Sbitany said, "However, every surgery carries the risk for infection and when we place a foreign body in your body, that risk is greater. In some women, scar tissue forms around the implant that then tucks it down to the chest wall, called implant contracture, and sometimes this can only be fixed surgically. If the skin is very thin and stretched, it can break open and expose the implant. The risk for infection often requires removal of the implant, to let the skin heal."

I had forgotten how many details are involved in breast reconstruction.

My head started spinning, and I again wished I brought someone along to help me write all of this down. I knew all the facts, all the options, and yet keeping them straight for myself was proving impossible. I clutched my phone harder, desperately wanting to make an SOS call to anyone . . .

And then I realized that I really had reached my limit as to what I could absorb, forget about remembering anything. Clearly, I did not want to get into further details about different volumes, sizes, textures, or shapes.

In the middle of the sentence, I interrupted Dr. Sbitany and said, "This sounds all good, and I think I will want to proceed with this plan. What do I need to do next, to get the surgery scheduled?"

Dr. Sbitany looked at Janet and replied, "We will talk to our OR scheduler and find a time for me and Dr. Alvarado to do this surgery together. Since this is not an emergency, you will need to give us some options for times that work for you. The only thing you need before surgery is to see the pre-op team so they can assess whether it is safe for you to undergo general anesthesia. You should plan to be in the hospital overnight and then with limited physical exercise for three to six weeks."

Then he asked me whether I had any other questions. When I shook my head, he stood up and shook my hand. Janet got up as well and said she would help me with the scheduling once I had made up my mind to proceed.

They both left the room. I got dressed and walked back to my office.

My office was just five floors up from Dr. Sbitany's clinic, on the seventh floor, so I took the stairs. Normally I'd have made that walk with speed and determination, but today I lingered for a while in the sterile concrete stairwell long enough to compose myself. Almost as soon as I opened the door, two of my clinical trials coordinators walked up to me with questions. I could not bring myself to stop and answer, but instead kept walking straight toward my office. Perplexed, both of them walked after me. My executive assistant, Vivian, was standing outside my door with a stack of papers under her arms.

She took one look at me and asked the coordinators to come back in a bit. "I need her first, urgently."

She unlocked my office door and ushered me into the room. "What's wrong?" she said. Since it was a Friday, it wasn't unusual that I'd be at the clinic, as I normally went to see patients who came in with problems. She couldn't have known I had gone to see a doctor myself.

"Did something bad happened to one of your patients?" she asked, taking my bag from me.

No longer being able to control myself, I burst in tears. "I have breast cancer and just talked to the plastic surgeon about my surgery!"

Vivian stared at me in shock. Then she turned back and locked my office door.

Vivian, a stylish Japanese American woman, had been my assistant for only a few months. Her calm approach to my hectic and often unwieldy schedule had been an incredible gift, but nothing like this had ever come up between us.

She sat down and said in her usual composed manner, "Can you keep your vacation and take the time to think it over? You could have some time away from it all and it will be great to have family around for support."

I had almost forgotten about our family vacation planned for the following week—a hike along the Inca trail to Machu Picchu.

Before I could answer, I felt my phone vibrate. Janet had texted me: "The earliest surgery date we have is in three weeks, April 10. Can you wait this long or should I try put you on the wait list for a cancellation?"

I showed Vivian my phone. She opened her stack of papers and pulled out my schedule.

"Three weeks seems perfect; it will give you time to think—and give me time to rearrange your schedule." Somehow her pragmatic approach did not come across as unfeeling but was just what I needed in that moment. A sense that this was just another project with an unforeseen deadline, one that would be over in time, too.

My phone rang again. My husband: "Hani Sbitany called me! How do you feel about this?"

Per the cliché "opposites attract," my husband and I are very different people. Whereas I worry but like to tackle problems head on, he is laid back and fatalistic. I knew his perspective would be invaluable and he would be more than okay to wait.

I texted Janet back: "Please schedule me for April 10." Barely three weeks away. I could handle it—or could I?

I turned toward Vivian, hoping she'd hear my silent question and answer affirmatively.

"I am ready for the clinical trials coordinators who need signatures, and please schedule a meeting with the team and the clinic staff so we can sort out the schedule and coverage for the next few weeks." I had gained back my composure.

"Please take the time for your vacation," Vivian said as she walked out. My natural tendencies would have me ask for an earlier surgery data. Following the advice I would give to any patients, I heeded her words and planned to take some days off before surgery.

The days before the vacation are a hectic blur in my memory. I vaguely remembered to do all the required preparations for surgery. I talked to the pre-op folks and had my heart and lungs checked out. My throat seemed to be in good enough shape to put a tube down it for the procedure. All set for surgery upon my return, I put some distance between myself and the medical system to reflect on what the diagnosis meant for me and what I really needed and wanted to do about it.

Chapter 4

Adjuvant Therapy for Breast Cancer:
Why Early Detection Is Important

W e had planned to go on a hiking vacation to Machu Picchu. Everyone was looking forward to it. With the surgery date now three weeks out, I knew this trip would give me the time I needed to come to terms with my decisions. Freed of the walls of the doctor's office, where I'd spent so much time thinking about life-or-death decisions, my anxiety and fears settled. Out in the open, I could put the numbers and options in perspective for now and in the future.

I had grown up in the mountains. Being in the wilderness with rain and rough beauty always gave me the distance and calm I needed to listen to a different part of my chest—my heart. Step by step, hiking up the Dead Woman's Pass on the Inca trail to Machu Picchu, I reflected on what the surgery would mean for me, what was important for me.

From a purely medical perspective, my choice was straight-forward. I was happily married, with children, in a very supportive home and work environment, so losing my breasts at this stage of my life shouldn't have been a major loss. At least, that was what my logical brain had thought, until my emotions kicked in.

I was plagued by questions: *Do I really have to do this? Is the ability to cure this cancer, and having peace of mind, really worth losing both breasts? Can I really go through this?*

On the third day of our hike, attempting to be rational in my thinking, I was reminded of a frantic phone call I had received almost ten years earlier.

At the end of a long day in clinic, with several complicated cases, I was down to one of the last patients, a fifty-five-year-old woman in long-term follow-up who had had breast cancer five years earlier and was doing well. We were chatting about her daughter's just being accepted to the college of her choice and how everyone was doing well. After five years, her breast cancer was fading slowly from her mind. One of my favorite moments as an oncologist is when I get a glimpse into patients' lives, especially when, after a diagnosis of cancer, life has returned mostly to normal.

My phone was vibrating and I didn't recognize the number. Afraid it was important, I stepped out and called back with a tentative, "Hello?" On the other line was the frantic voice of one of my oncology colleagues in private practice, Dr. Burton.

"Pamela, my daughter was just diagnosed with breast cancer. Can we come up and see you?" he said, his voice trembling. I did not know him that well, but from what I remembered from his profile, he had looked about the same age as me; so, I realized his daughter must be fairly young, probably around college age.

I pulled up my schedule.

"Of course, I'd be happy to see your daughter. Today is Tuesday; my next clinic is Thursday—would that work for your daughter?"

"We are already on the way to the hospital; can we see you now, tonight?" he asked, the urgency in his voice palpable. "My daughter is completely in shock."

Picturing an agitated dad racing up the busy Florida highway with a frightened girl, I immediately softened and looked at my watch. It was 5:00 PM. "Of course. Let me make some arrangements and I will see you today."

I went back to work and wrapped up with my last patient. As she was leaving, she said, "Thank you again for all you have done for me, but mostly for never wavering in your support that I can get through this." Heartwarming. And then she reminded me: "I still remember how comforted I felt five years ago, when you told me that very soon we would be talking about my daughter's college application."

I was finishing my last note when our medical assistant brought in Dr. Burton and Nicole. Although I shared quite a few patients with Dr. Burton, I actually had never met him. Glancing at the medical chart, I saw that Nicole had just turned twenty-six. Slender with shiny brown hair, she looked like a carefree college kid, not someone who should be in my clinic. Distress and worry emanated from her entire body.

Settling into an examination room, I grabbed a piece of paper and began as I usually did with a new patient. "Please tell me from the beginning, how did this come about?"

Her father started talking, but I focused on Nicole and spoke encouragingly to her. "Let me hear it from your point of view."

She told that she felt a pain in her breast, more like a twinge. First it felt like nothing, and she could not be sure what to make of it, but then within a couple of weeks she could clearly feel a lump. That's when she told her father. She happened to be home on summer break.

"What about any changes or scaling of your skin? Redness, skin changes or changes in your nipple?"

Nicole shook her head and looked at her dad with trepidation.

He spoke up and admitted that when he took her in for an exam, he never imagined it would be serious. But because it was his daughter, and she was clearly so frightened, he asked his partner at the office, a surgeon, to do a biopsy. Today the biopsy had come back positive for breast cancer.

He handed me the reports—invasive ductal carcinoma, poorly differentiated, grade 3, estrogen and progesterone receptor positive, and HER2 receptor positive—clearly an aggressive tumor.

Reading through the documents, I saw that Nicole's tumor was not detectable on mammogram—not surprising for her young age. She had had an ultrasound that showed a 2.8 cm lesion in the right breast and likely enlarged lymph nodes.

"Is it really bad?" Nicole asked, searching my face for reassurance.

It *was*.

Moments like these are among the most difficult for even a seasoned oncologist. The sorrow and empathy for anyone presenting with a newly diagnosed cancer never goes away, but the heartache and concern I feel when seeing someone so young facing this diagnosis is still so much more magnified. I steeled myself and smiled gently.

"It's nothing that we cannot tackle. Let's get a few more details." I asked her some questions about her breast health in the past, and she told me that she'd first noted the lump about six to eight weeks ago, almost apologizing to her father. It was only one breast, and she didn't think to say anything. She didn't want to seem like a hypochondriac.

Her father started to say something, but I quietly interrupted him. "It is okay; most of our patients don't think of breast cancer first, and clearly not at your age."

We then talked about other members in the family. Her mom and her entire family were healthy, and to Nicole's knowledge no one had had breast cancer or any other cancer.

I looked at Dr. Burton. "Any cancer in *your* family?"

He shook his head; his mom was fine and no one in her family had breast cancer or even died at a young age.

"What about your dad?" I asked.

His father had died of gastric cancer, but he was in his seventies by the time he was diagnosed and was the only of several siblings in a large family who had had cancer. I was trying to tease out whether this tumor could be a hereditary cancer, such as BRCA, inherited from one of the parents.

He looked at me and asked, "Do you think . . .?" He knew where I was going with this.

"Nicole, since you are really young, it is a bit more likely that you have a cancer that is inherited. About 30 percent of breast cancer at your age is linked to an inherited mutation. That's why

I'm asking about your family," I said, looping Nicole back into the conversation. She gave her dad a questioning look.

He continued: "Would it not be more likely that she had triple negative tumor, which is more common with inherited breast cancer? Her tumor is estrogen receptor positive, and HER2 positive."

"That is certainly true for BRCA1 mutations, but not necessarily for all inherited tumors," I replied pensively and added, "We will do genetic testing for hereditary mutations, mainly for BRCA and p53. The absence of a strong family history and an estrogen receptor positive tumor will make it more likely a BRCA2 mutation."

While it is less common, BRCA2 mutation–related tumors can present at a very early age. My youngest patient with a BRCA2 mutation was twenty-one. One is really never too young to have breast cancer; it is just rare. And if a mutation is inherited through the father, it often looks as though nobody else has cancer in the family or it even skips generations.

Foremost, however, we needed to get Nicole's cancer under control.

I sent her father out of the room so I could perform a physical exam on Nicole and ask a few more questions—ones I knew the dad of a law school student shouldn't necessarily hear.

Her skin and nipple were completely normal, a good sign, but the tumor was easily palpable on physical exam. I could only barely feel two small lymph nodes in the axilla. Everything else checked out completely normal. Nicole was quiet the entire time.

When I brought her dad back, Nicole pointed to the pathology report, indicating where it said, "high grade and poorly differentiated," and asked whether this meant the tumor was aggressive. Could I tell whether it had spread already? And would she need chemotherapy?

"Let's slow down and take one step at a time," I said. "The size of your tumor and the fact that it may have spread to the lymph nodes make it a Stage II tumor. This means it is curable but needs treatment. Breast cancer is treated very differently depending on whether it expresses estrogen, progesterone, or HER2. That's just short for epidermal growth factor receptor, a receptor kinase that is expressed on the surface of the tumor cells. Since you are really young and the mammogram did not pick up the tumor, I would like to get an MRI of both breasts to see whether there are other tumors anywhere else in the breast with the tumor or in the other breast."

"I will do anything to survive this, even chemotherapy!" Nicole interrupted me.

"First things first," I answered with a calm voice. "All with the understanding that you will survive this and there will a normal life after you get through it. The main goal of the treatment is to make sure that the tumors don't advance and spread to other organs. Breast cancer can only claim a life if it metastasizes and takes over vital organs. Treatment therefore entails two major parts: We need to remove the tumor from the breast and to eradicate any cells in your body that may have spread already."

Instinctively, Nicole clenched her fists and then asked, "Do you think my tumor has spread already?" Her innocent face now worried, beginning to realize the enormity of her situation.

Wishing I could confidently say that it did not and put her mind at ease, I answered as gently as I could. "Doing a CT or

PET/CT scan can tell us if there are tumors settling in other organs, but such tumors have to be of a certain size, and it won't be able to tell us whether or not there are tumor cells that have escaped and are hiding invisibly elsewhere in your body."

After a pause, she asked anxiously, "Then how will you know?"

This very question is the basis of adjuvant therapy—the part of cancer care that is hardest to wrap your head around. We just don't know in whom the tumor has spread. I was not evading an answer. For any individual patient, we can only talk about likelihoods.

For example, if I were to estimate Nicole's risk of recurrence with a typical Stage II breast cancer, I could only tell her the likelihood of its spreading for a situation like hers. From many years of research on women with a similar clinical presentation as Nicole's, there was at least a 60 percent chance that the tumor had already spread by the time that she saw me. Over the next ten years, about 60 percent of women with a similar presentation as her's would present with metastases. But it also means that in 40 percent of these women, the tumor has not spread and never will, even if they did not receive any further adjuvant therapy.

Nicole really needed to know whether her tumor had spread. Yet I had no way of knowing, with her sitting in front of me, whether she was in the 60 percent group with hidden metastatic disease or the 40 percent group without.

The discussion of the benefits of adjuvant therapy is quite complex and really challenging to understand, when the mind of most patients with a new diagnosis of cancer is usually just focused on survival. Even though Nicole might have a 40 percent chance of not needing chemotherapy, I could not take the risk of her being in the other group. I did not want to miss the chance to cure her and prevent her tumor from becoming metastatic.

The best we can do is use complicated calculation programs; I could then estimate what the benefits of therapy for Nicole would be. But there is one more variable that makes the calculations even more complicated: Adjuvant therapy does not work in everybody; it usually works about 50 to 70 percent of the time.

Going back to a hypothetical 100 women with a 60 percent chance for recurrence: 40 women would not need chemotherapy; their tumors will not spread. Of those 60 women who need chemotherapy to prevent recurrence, treatment will keep 40 without cancer over the next ten years—however, in 20 women, the chemotherapy will not work. Mathematically, therefore, only 35 percent of those 100 women will both benefit from and need the therapy.

In Nicole's case, the risk was high and the benefits would justify the treatment. The decision to undergo chemotherapy is much harder for those with small tumors with low risk of metastatic disease, and only very few patients need and benefit from chemotherapy.

Since we cannot be wrong and miss when it comes to chemo, an enormous effort is spent on better identifying who is at risk and who needs this treatment. Even more effort has been focused on finding better treatment strategies that may replace the current chemotherapy, improve its efficacy, and make it less toxic.

As I explained the goals and challenges of adjuvant therapy, Dr. Burton chimed in: "Since she is triple positive, we can attack this tumor by many different methods!"

"Thank god, I don't have triple negative disease; I read everywhere that they are so aggressive," Nicole added.

Nicole's tumor also expressed estrogen receptors (ER) and progesterone receptors (PR), which means her tumors were fueled by the hormones estrogen and progesterone. About 65 percent of all tumors are ER positive. About 25 percent express HER2, a protein in the epidermal growth factor family that makes tumors grow faster, and so HER2-positive tumors are more aggressive because overexpressed HER2 can cause uncontrolled tumor growth.

Only about 10 to 15 percent of all breast cancer is triple positive, expressing all three HER2, estrogen, and progesterone receptors, and about 10 to 15 percent of women have tumors that express none of these receptors.

Among support groups and advocates, triple negative breast cancer is indeed much feared. Almost all patients who present with triple negative tumors have heard some terrible stories about it and think they are doomed. This comes only from partial information, however. There are subtypes of triple negative breast cancer, such as the basal-type triple negative tumors, which are very aggressive. These are more commonly seen in young African American women and in BRCA carriers. And probably most surprisingly, obese young women may have a higher rate of triple negative breast cancers.

"But is it really good that my tumor is triple positive?" Nicole asked.

The likelihood of the tumor's having spread is influenced by many factors and is much greater with certain types of tumors. Still, there are many accurate and inaccurate beliefs regarding what might constitute a "good" tumor. From an oncologist's standpoint, there's no such thing as *good* and *bad* tumors, but rather, what we are looking for is a tumor that can be treated and prevented from spreading. For instance, a very aggressive tumor that is highly responsive to therapy and can be completely eradicated is much better than a smoldering, low-grade tumor that just keeps growing and is resistant to therapy. Even a very slow-growing tumor will cause havoc at some point.

The risk of metastatic disease and the option for therapy to prevent metastatic disease are highly influenced by the expression of the three commonly tested receptors: ER, PR, and HER2. ER and PR are in the hormone family, and HER2 is in the epidermal growth factor family with a receptor located on the cell surface. Over-expressed HER2 in breast cancer cells promotes uncontrolled tumor growth. Excess estrogens and progestin produced in women—or given as medication and supplements—can stimulate the growth of ER-positive tumors.

Much is still unknown about many other factors that turn normal cells into tumor cells and promote growth. In breast cancer, the expressions of these three receptors strongly influence the outcome, and therapy is directly linked to their expression. A triple positive test in Nicole meant that her tumor expressed ER, PR, and HER2, therefore giving us more options to specifically target these receptors.

"Should we do an Oncotype DX test?" Dr. Burton asked. "Maybe her test shows that her tumor is not very aggressive and she will not need chemotherapy." I looked at him calmly, and he continued, "I know, the test is not meant for someone with HER2 tumors."

"No, for her it would not help," I said. He was referring to a test now routinely done in women whose tumor is estrogen receptor positive. Such tests as Oncotype DX, MammaPrint, or PAM50 (and soon others), look at the multiple genes that are expressed in the tumor to tell us whether a tumor displays aggressive behavior and whether chemotherapy is needed. The expression patterns of these genes in the tumor specimen can distinguish an aggressive tumor from one that does not need chemotherapy. The major impact of these genomic tests has been that we now can determine whether a woman really needs both chemotherapy and hormonal therapy. The genetic patterns of a tumor are now considered more important factors than the age of the patient, the size of the tumor, and even the involvement of up to three lymph nodes. Thus, even a young woman with a sizable tumor and a positive lymph node can be spared chemotherapy if she has a low risk tumor by genomic assessment.

So, when Nicole's dad asked whether I would order an Oncotype DX test, this was partly justified since her tumor was ER positive. However, since Nicole was also HER2 positive, such a test would not be appropriate—having a tumor that expresses HER2 trumps all tests and means chemotherapy with HER2-targeting therapy first, and then therapy that reduces the drive that estrogen provides to the tumor.

Taking all this in was clearly overwhelming to both daughter and father. And toward the end of the conversation, it became rather difficult to explain the principles of chemotherapy in the level of detail I would have wanted had we only more time with patients.

The principle of chemotherapy leverages the fact that tumor cells divide faster than normal cells. Even though tumor cells may grow out of control, the way they multiply is still ruled by a finely controlled biological process in which each cell *should* end up as two identical duplicates. Before a cell can divide into two daughter cells, the DNA must be replicated. Many of the existing chemotherapies interfere with these steps and keep the cells from dividing or directly destroy cells. More recently, clinical studies suggest that women with a BRCA mutation are particularly vulnerable to agents that cause DNA damage, as tumors without an intact BRCA gene cannot easily repair damage induced by chemotherapy. Hence, most patients with triple negative breast cancer should be tested for BRCA mutations.

In Stages I through III breast cancer, three types of chemotherapies are used. Tumors that rapidly divide are very dependent on intact and efficient cell division and it is easy to see that chemotherapy may be very effective in killing such tumor cells. However, because rapid cell division happens routinely in many cells throughout our bodies—hair, blood cells, lining of the stomach and gut, as well as many other organs (such as the heart), and the nerves—it's not surprising that the side effects are often widespread and difficult to deal with. Therapy may also be toxic to the heart and nerves.

If a tumor is aggressive, chemotherapy is given at almost any age as long as the patient can tolerate the side effects. I think my oldest patient receiving chemotherapy was a very spry eighty-five-year-old who had very few side effects.

Many triple negative breast cancers respond very well to chemotherapy; the tumors just melt away. And if a large triple negative breast cancer undergoes a complete response to che-motherapy, that tumor is not likely going to come back ever. In addition, for patients with triple negative breast cancer, all treat-ments are completed after approximately four months, whereas a woman with HER2- or ER-positive tumors will require treat-ment for much longer.

When Nicole asked me when she would be done with ther-apy, adding that she would do anything—even chemotherapy—I barely had the heart to tell her, that in the long run, chemo-therapy probably would be the most manageable of all the ther-apy that would be necessary. She would also need a year-long treatment of HER2-targeting therapy, and then five to ten years of hormonal (also called endocrine) therapy. HER2-positive tumors are very aggressive and until we had HER2-targeting therapy had a very poor outcome.

In 1987, scientists discovered that about 20 percent of all tumors express a protein on the cell surface that makes these tumor cells grow uncontrollably; soon thereafter, an intense effort to find a drug to target this protein ensued. Within a decade, the first monoclonal antibody–targeting HER2, trastu-zumab (Herceptin) made was tested and showed promise. In 1996, when I began my fellowship in oncology, we enrolled the first patients on the trials with trastuzumab. It was easy to tell that this drug would work well and many patients with meta-static, HER2-positive breast cancer responded to the treatment for a long time thereafter. I still remember the excitement when the data on the significant impact of adding trastuzumab to chemotherapy for Stage I though III breast cancer were presented at the national oncology meeting in Orlando.

Since then, it has saved many more lives of women with HER2-positive breast cancer, and several more drugs targeting HER2 have been approved and added. One that was recently approved is a pill rather than an intravenous drug (my patient was one of the first to receive it during the initial study, in fact). This patient was a woman in her late forties with metastatic HER2-positive breast cancer. She'd been told she had three months to live. Since she was a dog breeder and cared for over twenty dogs, she told me that it was simply not feasible for her to leave all her beautiful dogs behind, including one prized pointer named Pamela. She pointed to my name tag and told me that I needed to think of a miracle. She and Pamela won several more prizes over the next few years.

Usually the HER2-targeting therapy is well tolerated, but Nicole also had ER-positive tumors; those were thriving on estrogen. The goal of hormonal therapy would be to starve her tumors of estrogen. This can occur by two ways: by blocking the receptor where estrogen docks in the cell or by reducing the body's estrogen production. The benefits of suppressing estrogen were described well over one hundred years ago, when in 1896, George Beatson reported that a young woman with extensive breast cancer went into remission after he removed her ovaries. In premenopausal women, removing the ovaries is still a commonly used and very effective way of treating breast cancer.

Alternatively, there are drugs to shut down the ovaries. In addition to the selective estrogen receptor modulator, tamoxifen has been the long-term hormonal drug of choice for young women. The introduction of tamoxifen remains probably one of the most significant medical breakthroughs in cancer. It was a drug that had really been developed as a contraceptive, but failed spectacularly when several women in the first studies got pregnant. It is still now, albeit very rarely, used as a fertility drug.

Aromatase inhibitors, such anastrozole, letrozole, and exemestane, which reduce natural estrogen production, have been the predominant choices for postmenopausal women. And while it was originally thought that hormonal therapy could be done in five years, now women are asked to stay on hormonal therapy for seven to ten years. These are many long years for someone being deprived of estrogen.

Nicole was twenty-six years old, unmarried, and about to embark on a long road of illness and recovery. However, knowing that she would do well, I needed to plan for the future and also make sure that at some point she would be able to have a child. I am not sure Nicole completely realized just how much she would really be asked to do when she said she would do anything.

For someone in Nicole's situation, still in shock from the recent diagnosis of high-risk breast cancer, a discussion about having children may have seemed very low on the list of priorities. Not bringing it up is a common mistake that has been made by many patients and oncologists alike. Over the years, I have counseled countless women in the same position as

Nicole. For her and them, the preservation of fertility when life is threatened seemed irrelevant. Too many times I have heard, "That isn't important right now!" Yet we know that five years later, many patients had suffered great regrets.

And because we would have to suppress Nicole's ovarian function and give her chemotherapy, she also was at risk of becoming infertile permanently. If not addressed now, her ability to bear a child could be irreversibly lost—but unnecessarily. So while Nicole was anxious to start her chemotherapy, I was also focused on arranging for her to see a fertility specialist. I knew we had time. Despite the incredible sense of urgency most cancer patients experience, the initiation of chemotherapy for breast cancer, unlike leukemia, is usually not an emergency. There should always be time to wait three or four weeks to protect a patient's fertility. And in the case of Nicole, it would take that long to complete the MRIs of her breasts, the CT scans, and the genetic testing.

The risks of the chemotherapy damaging ovaries and the eggs inside are not the only potential complications for having a child post-treatment. Even if the ovaries were protected from damage at the time of chemotherapy, ten years of estrogen withdrawal and shutting down the ovaries by itself can put even a young woman beyond the limit of her natural fertility—which decreases very drastically after the age of thirty-five. With regard to the limits of conceiving a child, the age of the ovaries matters, not that of the womb. With frozen eggs or embryos, however, time no longer poses a threat. A pregnancy using frozen embryos can be carried at any age and can also be carried by a surrogate.

There are several options for preserving fertility in this way for a young woman before she undergoes chemotherapy. One method involves stimulating her ovaries to chemically induce the maturation of more of her eggs. We then harvest and freeze (cryopreserve) them in a sophisticated manner. In the early years of my practice, a woman needed a partner for this to work because only fertilized eggs would survive. However, new freezing procedures allow the storing of unfertilized eggs. These procedures are costly and require intensive interventions and appropriate timing. Moreover, the patient usually initiates her ovarian stimulation on the second or third day of her period, and her eggs are harvested after ten to fourteen days. Ovarian stimulation in women with breast cancer can be safely done with tamoxifen or letrozole, and usually this results in several maturing eggs. The eggs will be retrieved with a small surgical procedure and immediately frozen. However, since the timing of this procedure is so crucial, it often means a delay in the start of chemotherapy. So it's important to start thinking of fertility perseveration as soon as a patient is diagnosed with any cancer that is treatable with chemotherapy. Despite these advances, for many patients, egg harvesting and egg freezing has been very difficult. This is due, in part, to the high cost of storing eggs and poor timing from insurance companies covering such procedures.

Still another method of preserving ovarian function is to suppress the ovaries during the time that the chemotherapy is given. The hope here is that by chemically inducing temporary menopause, the ovaries will be protected from damage that chemotherapy may cause. This method is much more contro-versial, less effective than egg freezing, and not really suitable for a patient with ER-positive disease, like Nicole.

I looked outside; it had gotten dark. Over the last part of the discussion, Nicole had begun shifting uncomfortably in her chair. In addition to looking worried, she now also appeared completely drained. Most of the first visits with a newly diag-nosed patient are exhausting, but given Nicole's age and results, this felt particularly harrowing for us all. And while her father had many more questions on the details of therapy, I stopped him and turned to Nicole.

"Do you have any urgent questions for me for today? I know this is a lot to absorb, but I am going to schedule an urgent visit with a reproductive endocrinologist, and set you up with the MRI. And then I think you should see me again in a week, so we can finalize the treatment plans." I put my arm around her shoulders and gave her a hug.

"Do you think you will be okay until then?" I asked before she left the room with her dad. It was a polite question that I no longer ask, since I now know that she would not be okay, even if I had the time to answer all her questions.

When the results came in, we learned that her genetic test-ing did show a BRCA2 mutation. And while her MRI showed no abnormalities in the second breast, there was a second abnor-mality in the same breast about 5 or 6 cm away from her origi-nal tumor. And there was an enlargement of two lymph nodes. All of which were cancerous. It had spread to the lymph nodes, just as she'd feared.

With the goal of shrinking the tumors before surgery, we started chemotherapy first and then, because of the BRCA2 mutation, discussed a bilateral mastectomy.

A few days later I received a phone call from Nicole's dad, wanting to discuss the need for a bilateral mastectomy in his young beautiful girl. He sounded devastated, clearly struggling with so many uncertainties about her future. How would she deal with chemotherapy? How would she handle the surgeries, the fears of dying from the disease? Most of all, what about dating and marrying after a double mastectomy at her age?

I cringed at the barrage of questions. Knowing him better by then, I knew he did not ask because he was crude but because he was heartbroken.

I tried to address that latter emotion I could hear coming through: "Nicole is beautiful and kind. Anyone who loves her will not care. And the ones who care are likely not going to love her. She will be better off without such individuals in her life."

My response came not only from my natural optimism with patients but from experience. Having seen so many of my younger patients survive and manage the long therapy and extensive surgeries with exceptional poise, I knew Nicole would take all of this in stride—rough in the beginning, and precious and profound afterward.

Now, more than ten years have passed since that night my phone buzzed. Nicole is a very successful lawyer, happily married, and gave birth to two beautiful children. Her husband is a gem and truly supportive. Meeting her at a conference at lunch, I was looking at a poised and mature woman with a full life, and no one would suspect the harrowing time she had gone through. I asked her whether she wanted to talk about the time of cancer treatment.

She leaned back in her chair and took a sip of water, then she started with a calm voice: "If I recall correctly, the treatment plan unfolded over a period of time as the various tests and information came back. Initially, I learned I would need chemotherapy, which immediately conjured images of incessant vomiting, sickness, and hair loss and scared the living daylights out of me. I felt betrayed by my body . . . after all, I had done everything 'right,' eating healthy and being an avid exerciser since my early teen years. I struggled to understand how I got this cancer and searched for things I could have done differently to avoid this fate. After meeting with you, I accepted that I needed chemo and that it was nonnegotiable, and began to steel myself for what were scary uncharted waters. I gravely lamented the inevitable loss of my hair—one major attribute of my female identity—and the permanent loss of a sense of security about my health and well-being.

"Then after the CT and other scans and genetic testing came back, I recall you discussed the need for mastectomies, but I think you initially left the possibility of single versus double mastectomies out on the table. I was devastated about having my breasts removed, but I remember crying tears of joy that I might get to keep one of my breasts, which felt like some badly needed consolation prize after a barrage of metaphysical losses and soon-to-be physical losses as well. However, my attitude changed after my first chemo treatment. The chemo was so brutal and left me so weak that I immediately decided to have a double mastectomy, because I never wanted to have to experience chemo or have another breast cancer diagnosis again.

"I cried at every single chemo treatment as it seemed to bring the chaos of 'D-day' (Diagnosis Day) rushing back to me, and sitting in the chemo chair gave me too much time to think about my reality. With each chemo treatment, I became weaker and weaker, and after four cycles, I felt so weak and exhausted that I asked my dad whether I was in fact dying and asked him to be truthful with me. At those low points, I looked forward to the double mastectomy because I saw it as a definitive step toward stopping this disease and allowing me to reclaim my life. I had accepted the mastectomies. After four cycles of chemo, I was so ready to have surgery that my friends even threw me a 'Boob Voyage' party on the eve of surgery. When I finally had the mastectomies, I recall being alone in the post-surgery recovery room as I woke up. It was so quiet and all of a sudden I found myself weeping, acknowledging the sadness of losing my breasts, which had been a conscious or subconscious defining attribute of my female identity, the loss of my health and security, acknowledging the tremendous fear and stress that had become part of my life. But the tears were also cathartic and were tears of relief to have those killers off my body, and in some ways I felt empowered that I had done this to continue my life and to give me a chance.

"Of course, I will never forget the day that you announced that all of the tumor was gone and the margins were clear on the pathology after mastectomies; it established a rebirth of sorts. I owe you and my surgeon both a great deal, not only as my healers but for being my champions and believing in me when I didn't. Your convictions allowed me to continue. And now here I am."

She smiled at me with moist eyes—which mine were now, too. Her words cut deep, and yet I was profoundly proud she had made it through. I was also highly aware that her description of her cancer therapy reflected what so many patients experience.

But there in the beauty of Machu Picchu, I remembered my words to Dr. Burton, as I actively directed my mind back to San Francisco and my own surgery.

My husband walked behind me, struggling with the hills. I knew the hike was tough for him. Unlike me, he was not excessively fond of exercise. When given the option of reading a good book on a sofa or donning a T-shirt dripping with sweat while on a perilous crest, there was never really a choice. He is the quintessential professor: his head in the clouds, his mind always chasing a new idea. There are few areas where he is not an expert, and where he isn't, he's surely read enough. We had been friends, spouses, parents, and colleagues for almost twenty years, and between juggling two careers and three kids, neither of us had had much time to question our relationship and our value of each other's feelings and well-being. Both being passionate oncologists, we have daily discussions and disputes about our approach to medicine. I so intimately knew his ideas about cancer treatment and prevention that I could cover his patients on days when he was sick—or answer questions if someone called when he was out. I knew what he'd recommend, even if I wouldn't have done the same thing. But now, he was not the doctor, he was the husband. I had no idea how he'd treat me, his wife.

I began to think more deeply about how he would feel about having a wife without breasts. Would he care? I had assumed that he was somewhat opposed to the surgery because he thought my risk of dying from breast cancer was so low, that the surgeries I had in mind were excessive. But what if he did not think it was medically excessive, but really could not contemplate the thought of my being mutilated?

With a pang of regret for my disregard of his feelings, I stopped to wait for him. Our two preteen boys were walking just ahead of me happily chatting with each other, most likely playing Twenty Questions. My daughter was walking next to me, holding my hand. At age eight, she was already a fine hiker who loved nature. I asked our guide to take the kids up the hill a bit farther and then let them have a snack. I sat down and waited for my husband. With my feet dangling over the stone steps, I looked at the misty sky, clouds hanging low. The rain had just stopped and the sun was coming out, a reflection of my mood.

These questions swirling around my head, I watched him walking up the steps of the Dead Woman's Pass on the Inca trail. Slowly he was taking step by step, his cheeks flushed and sweat dripping down his face. His raincoat was still wet from the rain.

"How do you feel about having a wife without breasts?" I blurted out when he was about to reach the steps I was sitting on.

He gave me a look of complete incredulity—how only a husband of many years could stare at his wife who'd just asked what he thought was a really stupid question.

"Do you have anything to eat?" was his response.

I laughed out loud and pulled a piece of chocolate from my pack, then handed him some water. After catching his breath, he asked me what I thought about Martin Luther's translation of the Bible from Greek into German, establishing the German language. I sighed.

In the scheme of the larger world affairs, whether I had real breasts was just not an issue for my husband. And frankly, remembering our time dating, all other such questions, such as "Am I pretty?" usually went similarly unanswered.

Free of all self-doubt, I stood up, brushed myself off, and launched into a discussion on the quality of Luther's translation as we continued our hike and joined our kids. I knew he would not be the person to go to talk about feelings, but he would always be there for me and for mine.

Chapter 5

The Day Before:
Preparing for Breast Cancer Surgery

We arrived home from Peru early Sunday morning, just two days before my surgery. That same afternoon, I drove to back the airport to pick up my dad and his second wife, Marietta. Their visit had been planned for a while, long before my diagnosis, and I really did not want to cancel their trip. I had left my home country more than twenty years earlier and family visits had been sporadic. I'd go home maybe once a year for a couple of days, and my father would occasionally visit. Usually, Dad and Marietta would come for a few days and then travel somewhere else more exciting than a hectic household with three young kids and a busy, frazzled mom. Relationships in our family were always a bit volatile. And so, with no wallflowers in attendance, it took a little effort to cohabitate in a Catholic-Muslim-Swiss-Indian hodgepodge of a family. After two decades of practice, everyone got along reasonably well, as long as we avoided any conversations about race or religion—and we had very diverse views on punctuality.

Moreover, they both felt they could be helpful to me in my recovery. With the exception of having children and minor sports injuries, I had never really spent any time in the hospital as a patient. And only in hindsight do I realize how much I had underestimated the impact this operation would have on me. I'd envisioned being in the hospital overnight and then having some time off so we could hang out and go on long walks. My mother also had offered to come, but my divorced parents were still like oil and water, and while I love them individually, both of them together is always a bit much.

Upon landing back in San Francisco that morning, however, I began to have second thoughts about the wisdom of having visitors at all. What condition would I be in? How would my dad react when he saw me after surgery? Would there be silence overall, or deeply probing questions into the technicalities of the procedure? I thought back to other times when my health had been at risk. There was my misdiagnosis of heart failure, when I was pregnant with my daughter. This got cleared up and we never spoke of it again. The horrific car accident involving my two sons, who both survived and recovered, thankfully. My husband's hip fracture. No matter what crisis seemed to arise, Papa was always supportive with actions, rarely with words. Mom usually conveyed I could handle anything. But thinking back, I don't remember ever letting on that I was having a hard time with anything—that I was ever in pain or found anything difficult.

My German Swiss father, not unlike my grandmother, is from a generation and a culture where feelings are kept at a minimum and expressed only with extreme caution. He never talked about his mother's breast cancer—at least not with me. Just as my thoughts wandered back to how little I knew about what my grandmother must have felt, going through this surgery having no support system to hold her up, I got a text saying they'd landed and were waiting for me outside the airport.

Of course, I was late. Again. Ah, well, the first discussion would clearly involve a chastisement of my timeliness, or the lack thereof. I definitely did not inherit this Swiss trait. As I pulled up to the curb, I could see my father's steely blue eyes staring at me in judgment. Once settled into the car, he said nothing but checked both ways for traffic and then motioned when he thought it was safe for me to proceed. Still, at forty-eight. On the drive home, Marietta cheerfully recounted details of their flight—how much she enjoyed the view of the greater Bay Area, and how glad she was to finally land—but Papa remained silent and I focused on the afternoon traffic. Later, we had dinner at a local sushi place and no one really talked much about anything.

The next day was Monday—one day before my surgery. While everyone was still asleep, I quietly set out breakfast for them, for when they woke up, to enjoy without me. I left for work.

That day, I had a full schedule in clinic. After meeting with the team and setting out plans for all the patients on clinical trials, I walked down to the breast care center. Knowing I would not be there for a couple of weeks, I'd allowed the clinic to be overbooked. The day's room assignment schedule for all the doctors who saw patients that day in same hall hung on the wall inside the medical hub room. Handwritten notes indicated which patient was in which room and the names of those already seen would be marked with a highlighter.

Per my usual preclinic routine, I stood in front of the schedule, preparing myself to tackle what would likely be many unforeseen events and emotions. Most of my patients had advanced cancer, so I never quite knew what the day would bring—what symptoms would have arisen or dissipated, what complications from treatment had developed, whose tumor had grown out of control. Hopefully sprinkled in there would some good news for someone who was on treatment—a CT scan showing that the tumors were responding to therapy, or at least stabilizing. And maybe one or two patients who were just coming to check on lab values but had otherwise no side effects and did well on therapy.

Tara was already standing there waiting for me. "The schedule isn't looking so bad," she said, forcing a smile. Typically, she would greet me with a lilted "hello there" and an impish grin. But today her slightly freckled face bore a worried expression and her trademark sparkling chatter was absent.

I didn't answer.

"I am so sorry," she said, reaching out to hold my hand.

"About the state of this schedule?" I teased, raising an eyebrow. "You should be; this schedule looks awful, did you go out and sent invitations to everybody?"

"Everyone wanted to come and see you!" she said, defensively, but I could see her tension dissolving.

"No, actually, this is perfect. Let's keep busy. You didn't really think I'd be sitting at home feeling sorry for myself today?

And please, wipe that 'I feel so bad for you' look off your face! I am not going to the executioner tomorrow; they will take good care of me!"

She grimaced, quietly searching my face to see how close I was to breaking down despite my invincibility speech. Over the last few years, caring for very sick patients together had brought us very close. Tara knew I would always try to make her laugh, especially when things became really hard. There were many shared moments—leaving a patient's room, leaning on the wall outside, tears flowing down our cheeks. In this moment, I could feel her love and sympathy extending to me this time, and it nearly undid me.

But that afternoon, I needed to steel myself. I needed to be a compassionate and composed oncologist for fourteen patients in the span of five hours. And just as important, I needed to make sure each patient left the clinic that day with the hope and confidence that they would be fine, so that I could continue to convince myself I would be, too.

"Let's go. Later I'll tell you all about the trip to Machu Picchu," I said, knocking on the door of my first patient. "Especially, about that guide you recommended!"

Before my cancer, I saw patients and their stories as *theirs*, completely separate from me, the physician, who stood unaffected and in control on the other side. That afternoon I realized that any one of their stories could become—was becoming—*mine*. And whether it was just bad luck, or the protective shield of the patient-doctor separation slowly falling away, every patient I saw that afternoon had a complicated and challenging story. More than one story left me deeply worried. A thirty-five-year-old lawyer had first come in with a small tumor and just DCIS four years ago. Against all odds, it had metastasized and spread to her liver and lung. She was a mother of three who, despite experiencing uncontrolled nausea and fatigue with chemotherapy, was still trying to keep the diagnosis secret from her preteen children. There was the sixty-year-old nurse whose lymph node removal caused such excessive swelling that it made her physical duties more difficult. The moodiness and depression from the hormonal therapy in my high school teacher, which also caused hair thinning, leaving her self-conscious and embarrassed.

As the afternoon progressed, I began to wonder where the patients were who maintained their normal lives and breezed through chemotherapy, with little to no side effects. Most every clinic had some of those. That day, after hearing each of these stories of quiet, prolonged suffering, I began to imagine what my breast cancer could actually feel like. Until now, I hadn't had any real physical symptoms and likely blocked off thoughts that I could be feeling sick in any way. I became more and more upset for the patients and for the first time even more so for myself.

Again, I tried to calm myself with all the statistical knowledge I had. None of these stories would become mine, I said. My numbers were different: My tumors were smaller, Stage 0, my odds better. I would have surgery and be done with it all.

Later in the day, I was about to step into the room of a patient whom I had not seen in a while; she'd been seeing her local oncologist and only checked in with me occasionally. Tara had started the visit, and I was ready to join them just as she stepped out. She looked rattled. She waved me into an empty room and closed the door.

"What happened?" I asked, thinking back about the patient's last visit. Tara usually was unflappable. It took a lot for her to lose her composure.

"I'm not sure!" she said, shaking her head in consternation, explaining that Ms. Smith had basically dismissed her and asked to see me.

The two had discussed the course of treatment over the last three years. Ms. Smith had been on hormonal therapy and doing reasonably well. When Tara wanted to examine her as part of our routine visit, however, she got defensive and flatly refused. She would only let me examine her, she told Tara.

I leaned back for a moment, pondering the situation. Tara was not a person who would ever incite spite from any patient. "I am sorry for you, but something must really be wrong for Ms. Smith to act like this. Shall we go and find out what the problem is?" I offered reassuringly.

I entered Ms. Smith's room and found her sitting defiantly on the examining table, her arms crossed over her gown. I walked over, said hello, and gave her a hug. My usual routine.

"How are you doing?" I asked. "It has been a while since I last saw you."

From her local oncologist's notes, she was doing really well. Initially, her tumor had been more than 5 cm and had spread to six lymph nodes, making this a Stage III cancer. Stage III tumors, or those that spread to several lymph nodes, have a much higher tendency to come back or become metastatic. After surgery, almost all of these patients are asked to undergo high-energy radiation therapy, regardless of whether they've had a lumpectomy or mastectomy. The radiation beams cover most of the areas under the breast tissue and the armpit, as well as the area above the collarbone, with the goal of killing any remaining tumor cells that may be hiding. Her surgery was four years behind her; she'd completed her chemotherapy and radiation therapy, and was now on hormonal therapy. I knew she was tolerating the therapy well and had returned to work. All the mammograms and MRIs had been normal and there were no signs that her tumor had come back or spread to other organs.

"From a cancer standpoint, you are doing exceedingly well. But I can see you're very distressed today. Can I help?"

She was getting more upset and took some time to answer. Then she looked up at me, her shoulders hunched over.

"When I saw you last, I just had my mastectomy, completed my chemotherapy, and was partway through my radiation therapy," she began, hesitation in her voice. "I thought I was doing well, except the radiation therapy made me really tired and my skin was pretty red," she told us.

Both of these side effects occur in most patients. Often the skin gets deep red and starts peeling, but this usually gets much better as the radiation therapy sessions stop. Depending on the person's anatomy, there are four to six weeks of radiation with treatments five days a week.

There is, however, one considerable problem—reconstruction is much more complicated if a patient has radiation therapy. I could almost predict what I'd find when I asked whether I could examine her. She opened her gown, and both Tara and I saw what was causing her so much distress. Our eyes met and we held our faces as expressionless as was possible.

A broad, jagged scar had spread across her chest where her left breast once had been. The skin next to the scar was pale and stretched taut over her ribs. Her left shoulder was pulled down and her arm held tight to her chest. I then noticed that even her neck was tight.

She told us she had undergone reconstruction with an implant, that initially her surgery seemed to have gone well and she was recovering. Shortly afterward, however, and in response to the radiation damage, her skin became thin and lost its flexibility. She told us that her implant literally stuck to the chest wall. She was so uncomfortable that the surgeon had to remove it. The area became infected and it took several months to recover—so in the end she was left with an aborted reconstruction but tight scars.

Since we had mainly focused on the notes and letters from the oncologist but not the surgeon, we had missed this part of her history entirely. I winced at how our superspecialization in medicine can narrow our focus to the point of blindness.

"Have you gone back and seen a plastic surgeon?" I asked anticipating her answer.

"No, I just couldn't. I know, the office called me back several times . . ." Her voice trailed off apologetically.

I reached out and took her hand, "Well, let's get you back to see a plastic surgeon!"

She gave me a dubious look. "Why? I don't think I can go through this again."

"Unfortunately, your situation is not uncommon. Reconstruction is much more complicated after radiation because the risk of implant failure and infection is much higher. Often, it only becomes clear months later that poor healing and scarring have negatively affected the implant." Realizing I had slipped into my doctor voice, I added a suggestion. "Going back and doing another implant may be difficult, but you could have a procedure that does not involve an implant but uses your own tissue—a DIEP or a muscle flap."

I watched her face getting paler but continued. "I know this means more surgeries and that's frightening, but there is a lot we can do here to make this so much better!"

"Do you really think all this is worth it? At my age?" She was sixty-five years old.

"Definitively," I assured her. "And I am sending you to a physical therapist to get you some relief from tight muscles, and the neck pain I suspect you have on top of everything else."

"How did you know? she asked.

I forced a smile, imagining the agony this woman must have gone through for the last months, for no reason other than fear, and how possible it might have been to make this better.

Once out of the room, tears welled up in my eyes. Would this be my fate after tomorrow? Tara must have seen how much effort it took me to hold it together. She walked over to the medical assistants and before I could go into the next patient's room, one of them grabbed me and told me I was urgently needed in the infusion center—where our patients get chemotherapy. It is not uncommon that patients have allergic reactions during chemotherapy and require immediate medical attention, and I assumed this was the problem. Without asking any questions, I grabbed my stethoscope and ran up the three flights to the infusion center, trying to recall which of my patients was getting chemotherapy and could be having a bad reaction.

Out of breath, I entered the infusion center and the charge nurse pointed me to the room in the back. I rushed in, looking for a patient, but all I saw was Caroline, one of our chemotherapy nurses, waiting there for me with a cup of tea in one hand and a cookie in the other. We kept crackers and biscuits on hand for patients, to help with chemotherapy-induced queasiness, as well as a boost for blood sugar and mood.

"Tara told me you needed a break!" she said.

I almost burst into tears. Overwhelmed by their kindness and by the rapidly rising anxiety about my own surgery, all I could think of at that moment was running off somewhere—anywhere but here.

A few minutes later, Dr. Alvarado popped his head in.

"Just checking in and making sure that we are still on for tomorrow?" he asked with his boyish grin.

"I wouldn't miss it for anything!" I replied, my voice a bit shaky.

He looked at me. "Good, so per doctor's orders, go home and get some sleep."

I drank my tea and had a cookie, then another. Feeling replenished, I walked back to the clinic for my last two patients of the day, for the last moments holding on to the idea that nothing had changed. As long as I was the doctor, I did not have to face being a patient yet.

Chapter 6

The Day Of

On Tuesday morning, I had to be at the hospital at 8:00 AM. No food or drink after midnight. After kissing the kids good-bye, we left the house without actually mentioning again that I was not coming home that night. Since both of us travel frequently for work, it was not uncommon that the kids stayed with the au pair overnight. But no matter where I was in the world, I'd always call my daughter before bedtime and check in with the boys. For this "trip," though, we had not quite settled on what to tell them. After all, we really did not know what would be the surgical outcome. My husband drove me in his cherished Volt, and my dad and Marietta followed in my car.

Stepping into the elevator, I instinctively pressed the button for the seventh floor, just to realize that I really had to get off on three. As we walked down the hall of the pre-op to check in, Vivian and several of my clinical trials coordinators were waiting at the end of the hall, all wanting to give me a hug and wish me the best of luck—and maybe get just one last signature before I went under and then would be gone from the clinic for a couple of weeks.

The drawbacks of working at the same place where I was being treated were more obvious now than ever. I sighed and my husband gave me the all-knowing look, not the least bit surprised that several people were waiting for me to attend to last-minute business.

"Seriously?" he murmured. I looked at him, shrugging my shoulders. After so many years of being married to another oncologist, we both understood just how unpredictable and never-ending the work in medicine is. But my clinic had run late the night before, I had forgotten to finish a few things, and had actually told the lead clinical trials' coordinator to come meet me in the morning to finish up a few more issues. I knew there would be a lot of waiting around before the surgery. Just in case. Like every other patient, I had to be there at 8:00 AM even though my surgery was not scheduled until noon. And right now I would rather do anything—sign all the documents on the floor, probably even help out in the cafeteria—than just sit there getting myself all worked up.

With an exasperated grin, I told everyone to hold their horses and that I would have time for signatures after I had been checked in. I stepped up to the desk—moving into patient mode—and was greeted by an upbeat woman with a broad smile. She took my name, and checked me in. After handing me a plastic bracelet with my name and date of birth, she walked me to one of the pre-op rooms. She opened one of the cupboards in the room and handed me a large plastic bag, a hospital gown, a pair of socks, and one of those ultraflattering hair caps. I was glad I had remembered to put on some mascara in the morning, lessening how featureless this hair cap made anyone look.

"Please take everything off, remove all jewelry, and put your personal items in the bag. Your family can hold all your valuables." Her instructions were very matter-of-fact, and I became painfully aware that for her, and probably most of the hospital staff, I was just one of many patients coming through that day. It set me wondering whether I made enough of an effort to acknowledge the personal aspects of the patients I saw, and I immediately made a mental note to do better.

Once I had changed into a hospital gown and was sitting on the bed, Janet came up and asked me whether I had taken any pictures.

"Pictures? You mean, in case I . . . don't make it through the surgery?" I quipped.

"No, Pamela! Pictures of your breasts, so that you remember how they looked later!"

I looked at her with bewilderment, trying to find out whether she was pulling my leg. Granted, I had barely any photos of our wedding, because we'd essentially eloped; but I realized in the era of Snapchat and Facebook, that was probably unusual.

"And what exactly would I do with those pictures?" I mused. Other than being part of my body, the artistic value of the depiction of my breasts seemed pretty low to me. Forgetting for a moment where I was, I laughed out loud and briefly allowed myself a comic vision of putting a picture of my breasts framed next to my medical diplomas. It did not last for very long, and then a deep sadness began to well up inside me.

It was getting real.

"It may also help with the reconstruction," Janet said defensively. It took her a while until she got accustomed to my acerbic sense of humor as a hopeless method of coping.

The sight of a second nurse with an infusion kit further unnerved me. At that point, I was still very squeamish about needles, especially those going into my own veins. Distracted, I said, "Okay, let's take some pictures, as soon as I am hooked up to the drip."

The nurse came over and again checked my name and date of birth. Next, she took my blood pressure. She looked at me and said quietly just for me to hear, "Your blood pressure is elevated. Quite high, actually!" I did not have to read the numbers for myself to know.

"Well, I am a bit stressed out," I mouthed back. "I'm having a double mastectomy, and in case you didn't know, you have a very big needle in your hand!"

She nodded, uncertain how to respond. A moment later, she put the needle down and squeezed my arm.

Meanwhile, my oncology fellow, working with me on a six-month rotation, arrived with a large stack of papers that needed my signature. "Sorry, just some last-minute stuff . . ." She shrugged apologetically.

Telling her to take a seat, I let the nurse finish with my veins. Expertly, she guided the needle into the vein in my left arm, and in seconds I was hooked up to a saline drip. A cold chill went through me. Why couldn't they warm these infusions? I was hot just a minute ago, but now I was shivering, as if a river of icy water had started coursing through my body.

As I finished signing the last papers and going over the next week's clinic schedule with my assistant, Dad and Marietta arrived and settled into the corner of the room—followed by Tara, and Debbie—our breast cancer center's head nurse—another pillar of calm and support. My husband had been sitting next to me, checking his email on his phone, accustomed to the waiting and comings and goings of the pre-op area. His phone rang and he started talking to the emergency room about one of his patients.

The scene in my pre-op room was starting to resemble a Greek wedding. I looked over and saw Marietta chatting with the nurse; then, a couple more staff members stopped by to chat together. Vivian returned with more folders, and someone came and brought me another blanket. Everybody seemed eerily upbeat, trying to engage me in conversation, which was even more alarming. As I hid behind last-minute minutia, the pit of my stomach got larger, ready to burst. A wave of nausea hit me. My father finally got impatient with all this bustle and said to me, tersely in German, that surely there must be other doctors in the house who could sign these papers in my stead. I grimaced but was secretly relieved, and told everyone to leave me with their folders but not to bring any more.

There are different ways of coping with stress and anxiety. Mine more typically involve some sort of intense activity, so I can remain aloof. Patients would tell me that they went to a silent retreat to prepare for surgery, but just the thought of sitting cross-legged on the floor and meditating vastly worsened my stress. I tried very hard not to think of the inevitable removal of my precious body parts.

I looked at the wall clock: 9:05 AM, almost three more hours to go. And that was if there were no delays. Without anything to do, this seemed endless.

Then, as if answering my prayers, a gentleman with a bow tie walked into my room, carrying a gray metal case. Befuddled by all the paperwork on my bed, he looked at me with a quizzical expression on his face and introduced himself.

"You must be our faculty patient. I am Dr. [. . .] from nuclear medicine, here to inject your lymph node tracer." I am sure he mentioned his name but my attention was focused on his metal case.

I had completely forgotten about this extra medical step, on top of the surgery: the sentinel lymph node biopsy.

It used to be that surgeons would remove ten to twenty of the normally twenty to forty lymph nodes present in the armpit on the side of the affected breast. The pathologist then would test these nodes for tumor cells that might have spread outside the breast tissue. Tumor cells that travel to the lymph nodes are more likely to be aggressive, and become metastatic. The chances of surviving breast cancer are not as good when lymph nodes have tumor cells in them. So, not surprisingly, surgeons originally concluded that removing affected lymph nodes would prevent tumors from spreading.

And so until recently, removing lymph nodes by a procedure called an axillary lymph node dissection was part of the breast surgery. Unfortunately, it left many patients with cumbersome and even disabling lymph edema and swelling in the affected arm. When I first started seeing patients with breast cancer, many women would come to clinic with a very doughy, swollen arm on the side where a mastectomy had been performed. For relief, they often had to constantly wear a tight compression sleeve from their fingertips all the way up to their armpit.

In the 1990s, several surgeons began to describe a method that would reduce the need for a full lymph node removal. This technique, called the sentinel lymph node mapping and biopsy, was pioneered in patients with melanoma and centered on the principle that a tracer, injected into or around the tumor in the breast, would travel to the "first lymph node," later named the sentinel lymph. This tracer could either be a blue dye (a deliberately noticeable color) or a radioactive liquid. The surgeon could hold a gamma ray counter wand over the armpit and identify the sentinel lymph node by the highest radioactive signal in the operating room. Initially, both methods were used; the blue dye, however, often left a colored tattoo under the skin, or worse, caused an allergic reaction. Hence, I got the radioactive liquid injected to find my sentinel lymph node and identify the one to be removed during surgery.

If the sentinel lymph node did not contain any tumor cells, then the rest of the lymph nodes would also be tumor-free and hence did not need to be taken out.

The arrival of the nuclear medicine man caused the room to fall silent. Here was this stranger leaning over my bed, wanting to inject me with a radioactive tracer, and all the people close to me seemed to rise in defense. He started to explain what he was here for, but staring at the needle in his hand, I stopped him and told him I already understood the procedure and its risks.

I had agreed to the tracer because we wanted to know whether any tumor cells had spread to my lymph nodes. Until all my breast tissue had been removed, I would not really know whether what I had was all ductal carcinoma in situ (DCIS) or whether there was actually an invasive tumor hiding elsewhere that could have spread to the lymph nodes. I was quite aware that the radioactive dose was extremely small, and I had often explained to patients that it is safe—mainly because it would be too dangerous for the surgeon and staff to stand around truly radioactive patients. Of course, I had also done extensive reading on the risk for lymph edema, discovering that the risk was really low, less than 5 percent lower in athletic and nonobese patients.

Yet this time, I began to realize that although the potential side effects from all the procedures were really small, I was having several procedures today. If each of their small risks occurred, they could amount to quite a lot . . .

Surgeries are definitely not for worriers—and the long wait did little to bring my blood pressure down.

Before I could express any of these concerns, he closed the curtain around my bed, wiped an alcohol swab over the area above my nipple, and injected a small amount of a radioactive fluid. Then he wished me luck and quickly left my room.

My thoughts about the radioactive material in my breast were interrupted by Dr. Sbitany and a group of residents coming into the room and pulling back the curtain. Looking around, he introduced himself and his team to all the people crowded in my room.

Then he stepped up to my bed. "I want to spend some time going over the procedure again with you. Perhaps it would be good to have everybody step out for a bit."

Janet and Tara nodded to my dad and Marietta and suggested they get some coffee. My husband said he wanted to go and check on something anyway. As I watched them all leave, I experienced a moment of panic.

Dr. Sbitany calmly described each detail. He would let Dr. Alvarado perform the mastectomy and the sentinel lymph node, then he and his team would step in and place an expander under the pectoralis major muscle of my chest. The expander looked like an empty breast implant, with a small reservoir that could be accessed from the outside with a needle. It would slowly be filled to the desired size with a sterile liquid over the course of six to eight weeks. Over time—three to four months—the muscle and skin would stretch to accommodate.

Then he asked whether I was ready to sign the consent form. This is the legal document verifying I understood the risk and agreed to the procedure. Consent documents are clearly necessary and specifically spell out what is going to happen. I've been on the opposite side of the consenting process hundreds of times, and I've always wondered how many patients are really thinking clearly when they have gone without food and drink for many hours and are strung tight in anticipation of this procedure. At a minimum, it gives the patient a chance to verify what procedures are exactly planned—as well as for which body site. And although they tend to stick out in people's memories, the risks can often get lost in the moment, so it's really good to read the consent form carefully. Despite my good advice, I watched most patients sign the document without reading it— and I was no different. Typically, I do implore patients to take the paper home and look for the side effects that could happen over the next days. It can be reassuring to know what to do in case of complications. And most often the consent form has instructions on whom to call if there is a problem.

"If you are okay, I would like draw the incision lines on you now," Dr. Sbitany said, and reached for the dermatograph, the purple marker that writes on skin and that doesn't wash away when the area is cleaned prior to the surgery.

He had asked me to sit up. Still shivering, I watched him silently while he made a complicated series of drawings on my chest, marking the areas for the reconstruction.

His voice was calm and soothing as he drew and explained, glancing back and forth between me and his residents. "This helps the breast surgeon to use the same incision for the mastectomy that is ideal for the reconstruction and lays the foundation for the optimal reconstruction."

He glanced up at me and added: "Once you are asleep and lying flat, this is much more difficult. We also need to mark the site of the sentinel lymph node biopsy! When we're finished, Dr. Alvarado will come in to say hello and make sure you are all set."

"Do you have any questions?" he looked first at me and then at my husband, who had come back in the meantime and was standing by my side, holding my hand.

"How long do you think the procedure will take?" my husband asked.

"Including all the preparations, she should be back in recovery within three or four hours—maybe sooner. You know we want to keep her overnight and let her go in the morning, if all goes well.

"Then you'll see me in about a week for follow-up, and the drains will come out in another two to three weeks," he added.

"Drains?" I asked.

"In almost every body, the tissue response to the surgery results in fluid accumulation under the incision and around the expander. So we place small tubes around the expander to drain this fluid. The drains will be pulled when no more fluid is produced—usually two to three weeks."

"When can I go back to exercise?" I asked.

He laughed. "You'll need to keep still for a bit! We don't want the expander to get irritated or infected. But I will refer you to our physical therapist who will work with you to advance your arm and back exercises, so you stay nice and strong."

"Arm and back exercises? I was more thinking of running . . ."

Dr. Sbitany's surgical residents, who had stood there quietly until now, all groaned in unison. The rumors that I was a passionate runner and exercise fiend was well known in the program.

"How about we talk about that when I see you next week?" he said, ever diplomatic.

Little did I know then just how painful these expanders and drains would be for the first two weeks, and how apt his advice was to "keep still for a bit." Or that I would do my physical therapy with clenched teeth, mentally imposing horrible acts of revenge on the woman who, after surgery, mobilized my arms and got my lymphatics flowing.

Another knock at the door, and Dr. Alvarado came in. He leaned over and gave me a hug.

"How are you, kiddo?" he asked with an upbeat smile. "Are you ready?"

"Honestly, the sooner the better! I am starving!"

"Okay, let's do the final check. Bilateral mastectomy, and right-sided sentinel lymph node biopsy?" He checked my arm bands and made the appropriate marks on my right arm, and handed me his consent form, listing both of these procedures.

While I was signing—yes, more paperwork—he talked briefly with my husband about another case and then turned back to me. "Questions?"

I shook my head. Having seen his work on countless patients since he finished his surgical training in Tampa, I knew I would be in good hands.

The medical teams left. I was worn out, what with the lack of sleep from the restless night before, worrying about what would happen, whether it would all go well, whether I would be able to handle this . . . It was only 10:30 AM.

Dad and Marietta returned and started to sit down just as the anesthesiologist came in. Ahead of schedule, I was up for surgery next—was I ready? With unexpected presence of mind, I asked him to check the postoperative nausea medication order. He looked at me and asked whether I had a history of postoperative nausea.

"I don't know, but I remember being really nauseated during a minor procedure with a sports injury. I get very motion sick and I had terrible morning sickness," I replied. As a doctor, I knew all of these were predictors for nausea after surgery. He nodded and made some changes to my medical chart and promised to pass this information on to the post-op team. He checked my blood pressure again, and started another IV for sedation since my blood pressure was still high. Once it was in, I looked up to say good-bye and saw, for the first time in my life, my father with tears in his eyes.

Dad came over to the bed and hugged me gently. "This is just not fair; this should be me, not you! You should not have to go through this at your age!" He struggled to keep his voice steady.

"I am going to be fine. It's so I get to live a long life," I murmured as I tried to reach out to touch his face—but my hand dropped, heavy—my dad's face, blurry.

It is the last thing I remember. The anesthesiologist had given me the sedative and then wheeled me into the operating room. Later, one of the nurses told me my father had stood there for a long moment with tears flowing down his cheeks, until Marietta took his hand and walked him out.

Voices. Someone was moaning. I realized the moaning was coming from me. Hands were grabbing my arms and legs and then my limp body was moved onto a different surface—something soft and warm. Someone lifted my head and put a pillow under it. As the room came into focus, so did an acute stabbing pain in my chest. I whimpered, but before I could utter any words, I felt a cold liquid flowing into my arm. In moments, the pain was gone. I drifted off again.

When I woke up next, the air felt light and clear. The pain was gone. I sensed someone standing next to me. Opening my eyes, I saw the smiling face of my friend Mindy, a surgeon and a colleague. I smiled back and reached for her hand. It felt nice, but my mind could not quite register why she was there.

"Is there a problem with a patient?" I asked, still not realizing I, too, was a patient.

"No, silly!" she chuckled. "I was operating in the room next to yours and heard you were done. So, I came to check on you. I hear it all went well without any complications."

I looked around the room, still not understanding. Groggy, I nodded. The room did not look familiar at all. My bed had guardrails around it.

"Do you have any pain?" she asked.

Suddenly, I remembered everything. I was in the hospital, not working, but waking up from surgery. Surgery to have my breasts removed. So that I would not have cancer.

My hands went to my chest. I felt the bandages, the tubes from the drains. I remembered one of my patients once telling me that it took her four weeks until she had the courage to look at her chest. Suddenly *my* chest started aching, but I couldn't tell whether the pain was coming from inside or outside. All I knew was I was not ready to deal with the reality of having lost what had defined me as a woman for most of my life.

I closed my eyes and winced. Mindy called for one of the nurses, who gave me more pain medicine—and mercifully, I fell back asleep.

When I woke up again, I was in a different hospital room. My husband was there. Sitting quietly next to me, reading a book. It was getting dark outside.

"Hi, you're awake," he said, standing up.

"What time is it?" I heard my own voice rasp.

"Just after eight. Are you hungry?" I must have sleeping for more than five hours after surgery. And hadn't eaten for twenty-four.

I turned and saw a tray with food on the table next to my bed, but it looked pretty empty. I grinned, my lips and face dry and tight My husband had already polished off my hospital dinner. The familiarity of such simple things—his eating my food while reading a book—eased the sadness that was saturating my cells, my muscles, my heart.

"A little, but it doesn't seem like there's any food left for me."

"Oh, yeah, that," he said, looking at the tray apologetically. "Let me order you something. Thai or Vietnamese?"

The rest of the evening was a blur. A few colleagues stopped by between their late-night rounds and chatted with my husband. My chest was sore, but the nurses gave me strong pain medication about every two hours that dulled the powerful, immediate waves. The surgery resident checked my incisions for bleeding—then emptied the bulb at the end of my drains, a small reservoir that would fill up with the reddish-yellow fluid leaving my wounds.

Finally more awake, I looked at the clock at the wall: 2:00 AM. My husband was peacefully sleeping on the pull-out chair next to me. I hadn't seen what I looked like under the bandages, but I was content. Still pleasantly lulled by the slowly disappearing effects of all the drugs, I decided that for the moment, reality could wait.

Shortly before morning, a nurse came back in and gave me more pain medicine. Fully awake now, the effects of the morphine taking the pain away, I lay there in my hospital bed and let my thoughts wander. *How did I get breast cancer?* Loosely associating memories, I was thinking back to a trip to the Field Museum of Natural History in Chicago with my son two years back. At a special exhibit of Egyptian history, we listened to a curator talk about a royal woman, believed to be in her early forties, who had multiple spine lesions detected on a CT scan. The expert told us the young royal likely had tuberculosis.

Looking at the mummy of this woman, and her solid bones and well-preserved teeth, I muttered under my breath to my son: "This CT sure looks like metastatic breast cancer to the bones, to me."

My son gave me *the look*—the expression all my kids give when I go too far into doctor mode in real life—so I restrained myself from delving into an argument with the curator about whether this was actually breast cancer or tuberculosis. I looked at the CT images some more and then at the mummy. Why couldn't she have had breast cancer?

We know breast cancer has been around for centuries, and is the most common cancer in women. And every woman with breast cancer invariably will ask herself what I had not allowed myself to ask so far: *Why me? What did I do wrong to get breast cancer?*

Like many of those questioning women, I never considered myself someone truly at risk—someone who needed to worry; but rather, someone who was immune to the disease I treated every day. One would think, what with my being around so many patients with breast cancer, that it should have been in the forefront of my worries.

Breast cancer is the most common cancer worldwide, making up almost a quarter of all new cases each year, and it has been slowly but steadily rising. One in eight American women will be diagnosed with breast cancer over her life span, with 230,000 new cases per year and over 40,000 women each year dying from breast cancer in the US. Most breast cancers occur in older women, but 10,000 women under the age of forty will find themselves with breast cancer—and this is important—breast cancer at a young age is more aggressive and carries a much higher risk of death. This is particularly true for black women.

There is much discussion why we are seeing so many young patients with breast cancer. However, contrary to what it appears, breast cancer is rising mainly in older women, with the highest risk after age seventy—while rates in young women remain fairly steady. To answer the question *why me?*—for many women, there is no good reason for having breast cancer. However, there are factors that increase the risk for breast cancer. Age is a risk factor—because simply put, getting older makes it more likely to have breast cancer. Other factors that have been suggested to increase the risk for breast cancer are the number of years a woman is menstruating, early menarche and late menopause, not breastfeeding, increased body weight, lack of exercise, alcohol and other environmental factors, as well as hormones.

All medical students are told that starting menstruation early and entering menopause after the age of fifty-five are risk factors, as well as being older when one bears one's first child or not ever having been pregnant, increase the risk for breast cancer. I have recited these facts to many of my patients, even while fully aware that if such risk factors are present, they probably only increase the risk of cancer by one- or twofold.

There are also misconceptions and confounders. Girls are not actually getting their period much earlier these days than historically. Looking at girls at the beginning of 1900, there was a slight decrease in the age of menarche compared to girls born fifty years later. However, a large study showed that the age of first menstrual cycle in US girls is twelve years, which has not changed between 1973 and 2003, and 80 percent of all girls start menstruating between age eleven and fourteen. However, this alone is unlikely to account for the increase in breast cancer during this time period.

Similarly, the median age to enter menopause is now fifty-one, which is higher in wealthier countries and has increased over the last hundred years. Entering natural menopause at an older age goes hand in hand with a longer overall life expectancy. Other factors in the timing of menopause include one's sociocultural environment, their smoking habits and body weight, as well as number of pregnancies and at what age. But all these factors may be either directly or indirectly linked to breast cancer, too, and breast cancer may have little to do with the age of menopause.

Even before I was a patient, I had struggled with what to do with this rather unhelpful information about breast cancer risk and preventing breast cancer. Life for the busy, professional, twenty-first-century woman is hard enough on a good day. I doubt many of us really have the foresight to carefully plan the optimal timing of our first pregnancy so as to prevent breast cancer, let alone control our menstrual cycles, be it their beginning or end. However, I did try my best to follow all the breastfeeding recommendations, another factor for reducing the risk for breast cancer.

As someone who treats breast cancer, however, I am more interested in risk factors that a woman might be able to control herself, as part of her lifestyle—such as obesity (particularly after menopause), regular exercise, and excessive use of alcohol. Clearly there are many good reasons to battle obesity and avoid a sedentary lifestyle. The obesity link to breast cancer is still not entirely clear. Obesity has a strong link to endometrial, gallbladder, and esophageal cancers; but surprisingly, is much less strongly associated with postmenopausal breast cancer, and does not explain breast cancer in younger women.

So why is almost every doctor always on your case to lose weight and exercise for overall optimal health, including cancer prevention? While there is no clear proof that obesity causes breast cancer, there is much evidence that women with breast cancer who lose weight and exercise live longer and do better. Reducing the time on the couch and breaking a sweat *frequently* has very significant health benefits, and probably not just for physical, but also emotional well-being.

One risk that has been hotly debated is the use of hormones, mainly estrogens and progestins. Per the outcries in medical reports and media, estrogen replacement therapy has gone from being the "fountain of youth" to being downright dangerous. The truth is probably somewhere in the middle. Estrogen is one of the essential hormones that define being female. Mainly produced in the ovaries, estrogen gradually decreases over years and drops abruptly when a woman enters menopause. Losing estrogen causes many adverse effects, ranging from bone and hair loss to difficulties with memory and hot flashes. Not surprisingly, many women would likely take hormone replacement therapy (HRT) at some point. There has been a lot of confusion on the use of estrogen for hormone replacement therapy. A large study involving over forty-eight thousand nurses suggested that in postmenopausal women between the ages of thirty and sixty-three, estrogen would reduce the risk for heart disease. However, in the same year (1985), the famous Framingham study that looked at heart health of residents in the town of Framingham showed that estrogens actually increased the risk for heart disease. The link between estrogen and progesterone replacement therapy and breast cancer has traveled a similar path.

Many cancer experts warned that, based on the Framingham study, estrogen and progesterone would increase the risk for breast cancer. The Women's Health Initiative (WHI) study, a very large research project studying the influence of estrogen on women's health and well-being, likewise suggested that there is increased risk of breast cancer for women who were taking combined hormone replacement therapy between the ages of fifty and seventy-nine. Thus, when the data from the WHI study was presented in 2002, most doctors stopped prescribing it for fear of causing breast cancer. However, the risk was only really considerable when taking hormones for prolonged periods of time and when estrogen was combined with progesterone. Nonetheless, a large majority of women stopped their HRT, which over the next two years led to a temporary decrease in breast cancer (as recorded in 2003).

This is a scenario where hype and fear clearly overruled scientific rigor and details, and for years many women were left with no remedy for their often extremely disruptive menopausal symptoms. A woman's life should not be wrecked when entering menopause, as a short exposure to combined hormonal therapy for those who suffer menopausal symptoms is probably fine. Moreover, the ongoing WHI study clearly shows no risk for breast cancer for those taking estrogen only. And if anything, there may be a benefit with regard to breast, colorectal, and other cancers, along with a decrease in postmenopausal bone fractures. For those women with an intact uterus, the combined hormone replacement should be of limited time, as there is a small but noticeable increase in heart disease, strokes, and breast cancer. As is true with diet, "everything in moderation and with good cause" is a wise general rule to follow.

One of the most important risk factors, however, is having a strong family history of breast cancer or a gene mutation that causes it.

In the words of one of my breast cancer patients: "There are seven first-degree female relatives on my mother's side and among us there only five breasts left. I was just born into the wrong family." Having a strong family history of breast cancer and having a prior breast cancer diagnosis increases one's risk by ten- to twentyfold. Much before we knew about gene mutations, we have known that some families are blighted with breast cancer and that many women in the family are diagnosed with breast cancer when much under the age of fifty. Often there are several generations of young women with breast cancer. But then there are those stories where it apparently skips a generation just to be back with a vengeance. It's obvious that there must be something that is passed on from one generation to the next. Many factors have been suspected, including viruses— except viruses would not limit themselves to just directly related family members. By the end of the 1980s, it had become clear that certain familial breast cancer was linked to a gene. The currently best-known genes associated with breast cancer are the BRCA1 and BRCA2. Having such a gene means that a mutation carrier may have a 60 to 80 percent chance of having breast cancer over a lifetime; and moreover, a high chance of having breast cancer at any age.

I finally dozed off again and stopped trying to find a reason for me to have breast cancer. I really did not have any risk factors, Maybe I just had bad luck, like so much of my patients who struggle to find a reason why they had breast cancer. The question *why me?* has been posed to me so many times. And it would continue to plague me.

Chapter 7

Hereditary Cancer and BRCA Mutations:
Preventing Ovarian Cancer

Three months had passed since my double mastectomy and breast reconstruction. I should have relaxed. Odds were that with regular follow-up, I'd be fine, but instead, that nagging intuition of mine came back. It got so loud that I couldn't resist much longer and headed to the pathology department. Without hesitation, I asked the pathologist, Britt-Marie Ljung, who was overseeing all breast cancers in our department, now including mine, "Can we take another look at my slides?"

If she was surprised, she did not show it, but instead requested my slides to be brought up and then sat with me at the double-headed microscope.

What appeared under the microscope was bizarre and totally unexpected. Interspersed among my breast cancer cells were other odd-shaped cells in various stages of becoming cancer—all surrounded by scores of lymphocytes that had rallied to my defense. This was reminiscent of something we see in the earliest form of ovarian cancer. But, it couldn't be—I refused to fathom that my type of in situ (still confined to the site) breast cancer looked just like the in situ ovarian cancer found in BRCA mutation carriers.

But that couldn't be right! It couldn't be BRCA.

Looking over the eyepiece of the microscope, I glanced at my colleague and friend. Was it unusual to have so many lymphocytes surrounding the tumors? Until now we had totally focused on the more pertinent facts: Are there really no hidden areas that contained any invasive tumors? And that this was truly still Stage 0 cancer. Lymphocytes are not typically mentioned on the standard pathology report. She looked at my slides and agreed: for a common Stage 0 breast cancer, it would be unusual to have the tumor surrounded by so many lymphocytes. Researchers have long known that BRCA mutation-patients' tumors look different. This is particularly common for BRCA1 positive tumors, and, to a lesser degree, for BRCA2 positive tumors.

Reassured that there were no invasive tumor cells on my slides, I was now consumed by the thought that this could be a sign that I was harboring a BRCA mutation. And like Nicole, I needed an answer.

My breast cancer diagnosis was in March, and now it was November. Reflecting back, why did I not get tested when I was first diagnosed? As an expert-patient, why did I not even think about getting tested for a BRCA mutation? The very short answer is that I did not really meet the criteria for testing and the test would have cost several thousand dollars were my insurance to decline to pay for it. The long answer is more complicated. No one recommended it.

Typically, the person to answer whether to get genetic testing is a genetic counselor. Before a 2013 Supreme Court ruling, Myriad Labs was the sole lab in the world approved to provide BRCA mutation testing. The out-of-pocket cost for this simple blood test started at $2,000 and was often much more; insurance only covered women diagnosed under the age of fifty with a strong family history of breast cancer. So, in 2012, at the time of my diagnosis, it was not trivial to obtain genetic testing to determine whether I had a BRCA mutation.

I made a formal appointment with Amie, our hospital's head genetic counselor, and discussed my fears that I carried a BRCA mutation. As with every other patient, she carefully established my "cancer family tree" and discussed all my family members in detail. As we spoke at length about my history, I could tell she thought I was I overreacting. And justifiably so: There was really not much breast and no ovarian cancer in my family. It was much more likely that I had a non-BRCA-related breast cancer, as is the case for the vast majority of all breast cancers. No one in my mother's immediate family had breast cancer. She did not have sisters, but she did have over twenty female cousins and aunts, and everybody seems to live forever. My mom's mother died in her early forties from colon cancer, which is not really thought of as being related to BRCA mutations. Then there was my paternal grandmother with breast cancer. In medical terms, a "strong family history" refers to having more than one first-degree family member with cancer diagnosed under the age of fifty. Since my grandmother was over sixty when she was diagnosed and not a first-degree relative, she did not count. The task of establishing my genetic risk was not helped by the fact that my family is small. My father did not have any siblings, and my mom only had one brother who had no children until very late in life. Without an established family history of breast or ovarian cancer, the likelihood of my having a BRCA mutation was estimated—by a sophisticated calculator that Amie used—to be less than 1 percent; exceedingly low.

So, would it really be wise to spend several thousand dollars out of pocket, to search for a mutated BRCA gene with a less than 1 percent chance of finding one? Despite the clear and logical response to this question, my genetic counselor let herself be persuaded to order the test for me because I was under the age of fifty at the time of my diagnosis, and my family was really small, but maybe foremost because I convinced her that I would sleep so much better if I knew that I did not have the BRCA mutation. It was my money, after all, and spending it on that crucial peace of mind outweighed all other logic. In my mind, I kept seeing all those lymphocytes around my tumors. I needed solid evidence of not having a mutation.

As Amie hunched over her clipboard, checking boxes about my history to find a reason to support my testing, I was reminded of Kate's case. Her father had had gastric cancer, although no one else in the family had breast cancer, at any age. We know now that it wasn't her mother from whom she inherited the gene. As with her family and in many other cases, the mutation seems to have skipped a generation. Except it does not really *skip generations*—the mutation is there, but since no one tested her father's gastric cancer for the BRCA mutation, it went unnoticed.

Amie repeated, "You know the test is not likely going to be paid for." We looked over the risk criteria in the employee insurance handbook, and because my risk was calculated to be less than 1 percent of carrying this gene, I would likely have no coverage. We did find a loophole, though: I was under the age of fifty, I had had tumors in multiple places, the other side of my breast was also abnormal. With these criteria there was a slim chance that I would meet criteria for insurance reimbursement, but knowing that I was determined regardless, she filled out the paperwork anyway and got a test kit. (Now the test can be ordered online and costs as little as $99, or is free at select hospitals.)

Once the logistics were out of the way, Amie briefed me thoroughly with standard pretest counseling—detailed information about what a positive result would mean, something that I know only all too well from my patients. As with any other test, it truly helps to be prepared and understand the implications of any result. In medicine, a positive finding or test result typically means something "bad."

The two BRCA genes have been most frequently associated with breast and ovarian cancers, especially aggressive types in early adulthood. High-profile celebrities, such as Angelina Jolie, Christina Applegate, Sheryl Crow, and Sharon and Kelly Osbourne, have recently brought attention to their breast cancer and the impact of a BRCA mutation. The mutation is considered rare, but it is still unclear how frequent the mutation is in general populations. The frequency for BRCA1 or BRCA2 mutations may be as high as 1 in 40 as found in Ashkenazy Jews, or much rarer as currently estimated in other communities at 1 in 400. Many researchers, including in our group, are currently testing randomly selected individuals without cancer to better understand what the true probability to carry this mutation is. No matter how rare the mutation is, a carrier is at high risk of developing a cancer that probably could be prevented. So I left Amie's office, reassuring myself that my risk for this mutation was actually still very low. Except if my hunch was right, there could be other cancers. . . .

Three weeks later, on Election Day, I was walking back to the office from the polls when Amie called.

"Hi, there," she said with a strained tone in her voice. "I'll be darned, Dr. Munster; you *do* have a BRCA 2 mutation. Can you come by so we can discuss this in more detail?"

Could I really have a BRCA2 mutation? If having a BRCA1 and BRCA2 mutation means having a close to 80 percent chance of having breast cancer, how could it be that I was the only young person with cancer in the family? Was the gene silent or did it really skip a generation? Or a more pressing question: From which side of the family was the gene passed on?

The answers to these questions lay in the mechanics of the human genome. Every cell in your body contains a chemical code inherited from both of your parents. In humans, this code, deoxyribonucleic acid (DNA), is spread over twenty-three pairs of chromosomes—microscopic, threadlike structures that are packed in a very tight bundle in the nucleus of all cells. Each chromosome has a long arm (e.g., 13q) and a short arm (e.g., 13p), and the two chromosomes of a pair are held together by a tie, the centromere. Along both arms, these twenty-three chromosomes contain more than twenty thousand distinct sections called genes, which hold and form the blueprint of all genetic information. Your genes dictate the traits that you are born with, such as your height or the color of your eyes. Of the twenty-three chromosomes pairs, twenty-two of them control all organ functions and guarantee their flawless performance. The twenty-third pair determines gender—it has either two X chromosomes (a female) or an X and a Y (a male). Each gene has a duplicate to maintain genetic stability and guarantee that the human traits remained preserved over millions of years. When cells need to divide and multiply, all required genes are copied precisely down to the letter, so no information is lost or passed on incorrectly. This is most crucial at the beginning when eggs and sperms divide—nothing must go wrong.

Most of the time, this process runs smoothly and nothing in fact goes wrong. That's why humans have been around for so long and overall have changed very little. As important as it is to maintain human traits, one of nature's major feats is to introduce variety and the ability to adapt. Without the possibility for genetic variation, evolution could not take place. Changes in the DNA are called mutations. Mutations can be beneficial or deleterious or just insignificant, and mostly happen completely at random.

A global mishap that affects every cell in the body is fortunately rare, but it can happen. This only comes about when a mutation occurs in a germ cell—either the female oocyte or a sperm cell. When the affected gene signals an essential function, any fault or mutation can result in such devastating effects as the gene no longer executing its proper function at all or only poorly.

In contrast to benign mutations, which typically go unnoticed, deleterious mutations usually make themselves known sooner or later. Some gene mutations cause severe problems from birth. These include mutations that cause cystic fibrosis, or the craniofacial (head and face) abnormality of the young boy August (Auggie) Pullman in the novel and film *Wonder*.

To safeguard against failures, most genes have duplicate copies. The genes that cause trouble before birth or early on in life typically need both of the copies of the same gene to be faulty—usually one bad gene alone does not cause the disease. As in the case of Auggie, both parents carried the gene (or POLR1C trait), but it did not cause any abnormalities in either the mom or dad, because in each parent only one of their two genes was faulty. Such gene defects are called autosomal recessive disorders, meaning the bad trait is suppressed unless occurring in duplicate. In most cases, there is no clear benefit of having a disease trait; it just goes silent. However, in certain circumstances, having the trait for such diseases as sickle cell anemia or cystic fibrosis actually helps a person ward off malaria or cholera. When one faulty gene is sufficient to cause a disease, the disorder is autosomal dominant. In the case of the BRCA genes, only one faulty autosomal dominant BRCA gene is needed to cause cancer. Therein also lies the explanation of why, in autosomal dominant genes, 50 percent of the offspring are at risk for BRCA-related cancers compared to 25 percent in autosomal recessive genes.

Certain genes like BRCA do not directly cause harm; rather the role of BRCA is to protect tissues such as breasts and ovaries and be their defense against mutation.

As we go through life, small nicks and damages occur constantly to our DNA strands. Each person has multiple genes that are tasked to repair such defects; but if they don't function properly—or if the very genes meant to protect us mutate instead—the risk of cancer increases; and so individuals with BRCA mutations are at a gravely increased risk of cancer to those organs. BRCA1 mutations on chromosome 17 and BRCA2 mutations on chromosome 13 are among the most significant of these cancer-causing (or cancer-enabling) gene mutations. But it usually takes time to cause cancer—and so most often these genes manifest themselves later in life and typically long after the women and men carrying the gene have already had children. Hence, the BRCA genes get passed on from generation to generation. Unless a cancer-causing gene also affects the woman's ability to have children, this faulty gene will survive for many generations. BRCA mutations can probably be traced back thousands of years, and there are even suggestions that under certain adverse conditions, nature may provide a Darwinian selection advantage favoring individuals with BRCA mutations.

It is important to note that the faulty BRCA gene puts a person at *risk* for cancer, but it does not mean everyone with a BRCA mutation will get cancer. The risk of developing cancer is strongly influenced by other factors in a person's life, such as smoking, alcohol use, sedentary lifestyle, and probably many more, most still unknown. At the same time, certain organs are at higher risk; for women these are the breast and the ovaries. Men with BRCA mutation, on the other hand, have an increased risk to develop breast cancer, but less than 10 percent of the men with the mutation actually get breast cancer. So, if a female is the

BRCA carrier and has multiple female relatives, the likelihood for cancer is high. In such families, the BRCA mutation is more readily recognized. Whereas if her BRCA gene got passed on by her grandfather to her father and the family is small, then it may look as if the gene had skipped two generations. Since not every woman with the mutation necessarily gets cancer, it's quite possible that the mother, despite carrying the gene, may not have cancer, or may get cancer later than her daughter does/would. Or, as in my case, if the family is small with fewer options for expression, it may simply be difficult to see the thread of the mutation stringing throughout blood relatives' DNA.

For the better part of the last century, it had been suspected that certain familial breast cancer was linked to a gene or genes. Proving it, and then developing a commercial test for it that could be used in every woman, was, of course, a different matter.

By the end of the 1980s, the mission to find the genetic basis for breast and ovarian cancer started in earnest. A worldwide effort fueled by lots of funding was launched on garnering knowledge and resources to find the BRCA gene. In 1990, a team from the University of California, Berkeley, led by Mary-Claire King, found that the BRCA1 was on the long arm of chromosome 17. A dedicated, true vanguard in her quest, Dr. King had studied multiple Ashkenazi Jewish families where many females in the family got breast cancer and at a much younger age than expected. Her research was in many ways groundbreaking. At the time of the discovery, many still thought that breast cancer was caused by viruses or other poisons; but she persisted in proving that in the high-risk families that she had tested, those with cancer had a change in chromosome 17.

Based on her work, the BRCA1 gene was sequenced by Mark Skolnick and colleagues; researchers at Myriad, the University of Utah; the U.S. National Institutes of Health (NIH); and McGill University—all of whom discovered the exact spots where the genes were faulty and pinpointed the changes in the nucleotide sequence. The BRCA1 gene is located in a specific section on chromosomes 17.

As for any DNA, the blueprint for BRCA 1 and 2 is coded in sets of three. In BRCA mutations, rather than having a flawless series of preset three nucleotides, all of a sudden a letter is either dropped or inserted. This mistake can be anywhere in those almost six thousand nucleotides that the BRCA gene is made of. This then changes the sequence of all subsequent three-pairs, and the BRCA protein can no longer be properly expressed.

So far, more than one thousand different mutations in the BRCA genes have already been found. This is one of the reasons that genetic testing has been complicated, as finding a mutation requires the close analysis of thousands of gene sequences and all their possible variants.

If a mutation causes a loss of the BRCA protein or a nonfunctional protein, it is considered a *deleterious* or *pathogenic* mutation—words that cause a gasp every time I see them on a patient's report. Not all mutations lead to malfunction of the gene; if the letters match up, the mutation is harmless and goes unnoticed, and we call it *likely benign*. However, one category of mutations that lead to much heartache are those that are called *variants of unknown significance* (VUS), the medical term for "no one knows what to do with it," and for which we're not sure whether they cause cancer or not.

After the discovery of the BRCA1 gene, it quickly became clear that there had to be another gene involved. Looking at families with many breast cancer cases that did not carry the BRCA1 gene led to the discovery of the BRCA2 gene in 1994. BRCA2 was linked to chromosome 13, and a year later, that gene was sequenced. A neck-to-neck race ensued between UK researchers, led by Alan Ashworth and Michael Stratton at the Institute for Cancer Research and the Sanger Centre, who were publishing the results of their findings, and the researchers at Myriad Genetics, one of the early companies devoted to developing and commercializing a blood test for the BRCA gene. Each faction wanted to lay claim to the discovery of BRCA2—a fight that was ultimately won by Myriad, as the company already held the patents protecting the BRCA1 and BRCA2 gene and their testing, making Myriad the only laboratory to be able to conduct the BRCA test on women. The cost was between $2,000 and $6,000, reimbursed by insurance companies under only the most stringent conditions, and thus unaffordable for most patients. That was at least one of the reasons that I, and so many patients, did not get tested earlier.

When the Supreme Court ruled against the patenting of naturally occurring genes in 2013, the monopoly for BRCA1 and BRCA2 and other gene testing held by only one company for almost twenty years was immediately broken. With gene testing now being made available by several companies, the costs for gene testing have decreased drastically to as low as $100, and many more genes causing cancer are being tested for. BRCA testing is now less a matter of cost but more a medical-scientific and emotional question: Who should get tested, and if so when is the right time? We are still very far off from broadly testing general populations without cancer, and most men from BRCA families with cancer still don't get tested. We can only hope that BRCA gene testing will become part of regular care in patients and families with breast cancer, as knowing about the mutation has a great impact on their lives.

Before I really had time to reflect on Amie's news, I got another call. It was the frantic voice of a researcher telling me that our mutual colleague and husband of my best friend, Mary, had just been called into surgery. Henry had been waiting months for a liver transplant, and this morning one had become available. I went straight to the transplant unit to be with my friend. As we sat there and worried about him, I tried to put the thought of any BRCA cancer in my future in perspective. Having this mutation put me at risk for cancer, but it did not mean I had cancer. As I was waiting with Mary, sitting in the surgical waiting room for Henry to pull through, I thought about how relative most events in life were. Compared to the immediate danger of death my friend was in today, and the often imminent risk of dying for my patients (most are diagnosed with advanced cancer), I was actually given a chance to take precautions before having another cancer. Slowly adjusting to the news, I calmed down and spent the next few hours reassuring my friend that Henry would be fine. We heard the wonderful news that Henry had not only made it through the surgery, but that the new liver was working properly as well. Mary and I hugged, and I went home.

Still ecstatic that my friend and colleague had survived his procedure, it started to sink in that my personal brush with the cancer world was not yet over. It was November 6, and by the time I left the hospital, it was dark and a cold breeze had picked up. Shivering, I stood at the crosswalk to the parking garage and waited for the light to turn green. A nurse from the oncology ward passed me and said hello with her usual smile. She looked at me and quickly walked away. It was then when I realized my cheeks were wet, finally releasing all the emotions I'd been holding inside all day.

Amie's words from earlier that morning echoed in my mind, ". . . you *do* have a BRCA2 mutation."

I don't remember what I said in return or the whole rest of the conversation; my mind had shut off after her first sentence. I do remember feeling a sense of relief that comes with knowing that your gut instinct had been right. Not surprisingly, I felt an overwhelming sense of exoneration. Even three months since my breast reconstruction, a decision I really knew was right for me, in the back of my head were always the voices of some of my surgical colleagues: "There's no medical reason to do this . . . you are overreacting . . . you can keep the other breast . . . don't give up a central part of your being a woman."

From a purely rational, statistical perspective, and looking at population health in general, they were right. Stage 0 breast cancer has the highest likelihood of survival—and in many or most women, the surgeries are probably not needed. If we just had a way to surely know who these lucky women are, so much pain could be avoided. In contrast, in a woman with a hereditary cancer mutation, mastectomies actually do save lives. Several studies have shown that prophylactic (preventative) mastectomies, more precisely called risk-reducing mastectomies, in women with BRCA mutations actually do extend life and drastically reduce the risk for more cancers in later years. Not only does the BRCA carrier have about a 60 to 70 percent higher risk of having one bout of breast cancer—but 20 to 40 percent of women with BRCA mutations will develop a second cancer in the same or opposite breast.

While listening to Amie going on about what having a BRCA mutation means, one of my immediate thoughts was how glad I was that I had chosen a double mastectomy even when it was not then considered necessary. I had rationalized that I had done the right thing from a medical standpoint, but it was still very difficult emotionally. Learning about my mutation for the first time banished those insecurities and made me feel justified again. I *had* done the right thing, and now I had the proof my brain needed.

Of course, now I wish I had gotten tested when I was first diagnosed, which could have saved myself the agony of the decision-making. Had I known about my mutation, the decision on the bilateral mastectomy would have been very straightforward. Fortunately, now the procedure is much more broadly covered by insurance and costs as little as $99 out of pocket. All you do is spit into a tube; we don't even need to do a blood test anymore. Doctors and patients today shouldn't hesitate to test any woman for BRCA and other mutations that can cause an increased risk for cancer if it will help with surgical decisions, or if it would in any way alter the treatment.

But my relief at being able to prevent future cancer did not last long. Very quickly I began to realize that I was now at risk for, or possibly already could have ovarian cancer. The early warning signs are unfortunately pretty vague, including bloating, abdominal pain, and digestive changes that most people experience on a regular basis without their being caused by cancer. Now, I couldn't help wondering whether I did have any of those symptoms.

Another cold, wet breeze hit my face. I looked up and realized I had walked in the opposite direction of our office; sighing, I turned around and walked up the hill to the parking garage. Once in my car, I turned on the radio and listened to the daily news on NPR, compartmentalizing the other, life-changing news I'd received that day. Years of training as an oncologist and having given sad news countless times, I had learned to place overwhelming facts in a separate part of my brain and lock them away for a bit. It does not work for very long, but for the time being, I switched gears and focused on other things of life. The traffic was heavier than usual on my way home. Obama had been reelected.

Although my fuel tank was half full, I pulled over after about twenty minutes' driving, bought gas, and then picked up groceries for dinner and the kids' after-school snacks. I made a good faith effort during dinner that night. My husband, who is always a steady voice of reason, had so repeatedly assured me that I could not have a BRCA mutation. Intuitively I knew that this came from a place of self-protection and worry. Even now, knowing about the results of the test, I could not yet talk about this new piece in my medical puzzle at home—I couldn't stand the thought of bringing more distress to the family. Since my results had come back sooner than anticipated, I could keep this to myself for a bit longer.

Doing so meant having ample space to really sort out what this finding meant for the future—for me and beyond me. I was forty-eight years old, fit, healthy, a passionate oncologist, and now with one of the most feared cancer genes in my practice and in general. My risk now for having ovarian cancer was about 20 to 40 percent—and I had a higher risk of developing pancreatic cancer. Would I be able to continue working in a field where I see patients die of cancer that I am at risk for and not be consumed with worry? Would I completely fall apart whenever I saw patients present with a second or third BRCA-related cancer, or when patients came in with very unusual cancers associated with BRCA2?

But it also had detrimental effects for my family. My beautiful eight-year-old daughter had just watched me go through a double mastectomy and reconstruction. Now she would have to see me go through more surgery and endless cancer screenings. I had to live with the knowledge that there was a 50 percent chance my gene got passed on to her and my fate might be hers as well. And what about my two boys who could also carry this gene? Their cancer risk would be for prostate, pancreatic, and even breast cancer. Suddenly, bits of my childhood came together and made more sense—the death of my great-grandmother at age twenty-nine, from a cause no one talked about. Why my grandmother had survived her breast cancer, only to die in later years of pancreatic cancer.

All my life I have hated November. The days are already short and gloomy, and so receiving this bad news made this month worse for me. Over the next few days, the reality of needing to consider another surgery to prevent cancer slowly set in.

Ovarian cancer is the second most common cancer with BRCA mutations. The risk is much higher for women with BRCA1 mutations, and it occurs earlier in life. Ovarian cancer with BRCA2 is less common and usually does not start until after age fifty; there's about a 20 percent risk by age seventy. Since I was not yet fifty and had a BRCA2 mutation, I might be all right for a bit.

I could feel safe to wait to remove my ovaries and fallopian tubes after I turned fifty. However, research also shows that in patients undergoing a prophylactic surgery to remove the ovaries to prevent ovarian cancer, unsuspected ovarian cancer was found in a 2 to 3 percent chance during that surgery. Until now and as a doctor, I interpreted this to mean that there is 97 percent chance of being cancer-free. It was a fact I thought should be reassuring to patients. But well supported as they may be, these numbers feel very different and anything but reassuring when it is your cancer—in your body and not just on paper. No matter how much we quote and practice by statistics, numbers and probabilities rarely impress the individual sitting in the clinic with me. I had seen over years in practice how challenging it is for someone to truly understand risk when it pertains to oneself, and now I got to experience that confusion myself.

Now on the other side of the conversation, I saw the 97 percent chance I was cancer-free as a 3 percent chance I would have it. After all, my chance of having breast cancer in the first place was less than 1 percent the year I turned forty-eight. According to charts and records, my chance of having a BRCA mutation had also been less than 1 percent. Understandably, my confidence in the high probability of a good outcome had been completely eroded.

For much of my treatment, being an oncologist had been an advantage, but it has many drawbacks. A 3 percent risk is really not that much; however, week after week at my clinic I hear the stories of patients who had a very small risk for something bad to happen. Just in the very week of my BRCA test, I saw a young patient who came to see me for her very advanced ovarian cancer with a BRCA1 mutation.

Marcia had just turned forty and was in the midst of raising her two children and gaining traction in her career as an English professor at Berkeley. When she was feeling bloated, she shrugged it off as something women just have, probably "stress." As it became more frequent, she talked to her primary care doctor about it. They discussed many different ways of dealing with stress and she started doing more exercise. Eight months later, coming home from a late dinner, she noticed how much her abdomen was protruding. Staving off a short wave of panic over whether she could be pregnant, she chided herself for not noticing this weight gain until now.

A couple of days later, she toppled over in pain, had emergency surgery, and was found to have advanced Stage IV ovarian cancer. She has been on various forms of chemotherapy and investigational drugs for the last eighteen years. About six years ago, she had finally found out she had a BRCA1 mutation. If she had known about her BRCA mutation earlier, her fate could have been averted. But like me, she had no known family history of breast and ovarian cancer, so there was no reason for early screening or even risk-reducing measures—removing her ovaries before she had cancer.

I tried to keep Madelaine out of my thoughts as I began to wrap my head around more surgery. So far, I'd acted on each of my diagnoses despite their having a very low probability. I'd made it through two surgeries and was physically almost completely recovered. My husband was worried about how well I would handle a third surgery within a year; he wanted me to take some more time to recover, to wait and let the odds stay on our side. My former mentor, Dr. David Spriggs, an ovarian cancer specialist seeing BRCA patients in New York, had an imminently practical approach. He knew that since I was done having babies, I had no reason to hold onto my ovaries and would never forgive myself if I delayed preventive surgery and, in the meantime, was diagnosed. And he did point out reassuringly that menopause was not that far off at age forty-eight, so my suffering would be short.

All I could think of was waking up from surgery, and the surgeon standing at my bedside with a sad smile, telling me he found ovarian cancer. None of the reassurances from the medical team, nor the favorable statistics, would let me rest until I had the report from the pathologist, showing no cancer in my surgical specimen.

It would be nice to delay the surgery for a couple more years, and not go into early menopause, but would I really be able to sleep and not worry during the time I was waiting for the inevitable surgery?

The repercussions of ovarian cancer are a lot more frightening than breast cancer. It remains one the most difficult cancers for women to deal with because there are no really good options for screening. For any women with a BRCA mutation, having a prophylactic mastectomy reduces the risk of breast cancer by over 99 percent. If that route isn't possible for whatever reason, intense screening with mammogram, MRIs, and self-exams are highly effective at reducing risk. There's also the fact that most breast cancers are found at an early stage, either by finding a lump or showing up on imaging, and we have highly effective therapy for early-stage breast cancer, with a high cure rate.

Taking chances with ovarian cancer is more likely to be fatal. Like breast and most other cancers, ovarian cancer found at an early stage can be successfully treated. Except that rarely happens. For ovarian cancer, there are no definitive early warning signs, no good screening methodology, no matter what the stage. Still today, less than 50 percent of women diagnosed with ovarian cancer survive five years, compared to almost 90 percent of women diagnosed with a new breast cancer.

My research colleague, Victoria, was a rare case of early detection. She had a fibroid removed and by sheer chance her surgeon found a small mass in one of her ovaries.

She told me that her fibroid surgery had gone very smoothly and that as she was preparing to go home; she felt so good that she finalized plans to go to the opera the following day. Her surgeon came in and they were talking a bit about opera when Victoria noted that the surgeon "seemed a bit off." After some more small talk, the surgeon broke the news: She told Victoria that she was "truly surprised, but we found a small area of cancer in one of the ovaries." Victoria would need to be referred to a specialist—a gynecological oncologist, as the general gynecological surgeon typically doesn't perform such complex surgery as what's required for ovarian cancer.

Victoria was discharged from the hospital that day with her second cancer and much uncertainty as to whom to see next. Devastated. As a cancer researcher she knew exactly what this meant: extensive surgery and chemotherapy for at least six months. It had come just a year after being diagnosed with breast cancer at just fifty-one years old. Like me, she had DCIS. She was treated with a lumpectomy on the left breast and then had to undergo six weeks of radiation therapy. After that, she was supposed to be treated with tamoxifen for five years. However, before she got started with tamoxifen, she saw her gynecologist had ordered an ultrasound of her uterus because of irregular bleeding. Fortunately for her, this ultrasound found the fibroids, and by coincidence the fibroid surgery detected the 1 cm cancer in the ovary. Without this, they likely wouldn't have done any such screenings: She had no family history of breast and ovarian cancer, so the risk seemed null. Her mother had died in her nineties of old age, but looking at her family history more carefully revealed the tell-tale sign for a BRCA mutation. Her father had died of pancreatic cancer when he was only fifty-four. Now that she had been diagnosed with both breast and ovarian cancer within a year, her gynecologist immediately got her tested for a BRCA mutation. It was no big surprise that it came back positive. Hers was BRCA2, which causes ovarian cancer, fallopian tube cancer, and primary peritoneal cancer less likely than a BRCA2 mutation. She was lucky in one respect—that her tumor was discovered at an early stage and her survival after treatment was therefore much higher. Had she been tested even sooner, though, at the time of her DCIS diagnosis, she may have been spared extensive abdominal surgery and chemotherapy.

After talking to friends and experts, she found a surgeon and oncologist team with the qualifications she needed. The pelvic ultrasound she had prior to surgery still indicated she had Stage I ovarian cancer. The tumor seemed to be confined to her ovary and had not yet spread. However, only an extensive surgical exploration could prove this. To make sure that Victoria had the best chance for survival, the cancer had to be staged properly and as much tumor as much as possible had to be removed. The evaluation of the staging, or extent, of ovarian cancer can only be done by visually looking at the cancer during the surgery and then the tissue has to be further evaluated by a trained pathologist. Diligently, the surgical team removed both of Victoria's ovaries, both fallopian tubes, and the omentum (a layer of fatty tissue that lines the abdominal contents and covers and supports the intestines and organs in the lower abdominal area). Very frequently such peritoneal implant tumors, which grow in lumps along the lining of the abdomen, produce excessive fluid that can seep into the abdominal cavity. This is why women can have massive fluid collections in the abdomen that make their abdomen look swollen or even pregnant. Frequently, ovarian cancer metastases wrap themselves around the bowels and cause blockages that require surgery. In Victoria's case, the cancer had not spread to this layer or settled elsewhere, as is only all too common for ovarian cancer. The pathologist had checked all her tissues for tumor, as well as the fluid in the abdomen, and found no tumor outside the ovary, but just a few cells in the pelvic fluid.

Victoria's cancer was still Stage I, but since the tumor looked aggressive, she began six months of chemotherapy within three weeks' time.

I met Victoria at a research conference and we shared our experience with BRCA mutations. Spending some time with her at dinner, I got a good sense just how difficult it was for her to maneuver her care. She had many very good questions for me.

"Should not every doctor do a family history in a case like mine, and put two and two together considering BRCA? My father died at fifty-four and I was barely over fifty with breast cancer—could it have been any clearer?" she asked me with reproach in her eyes and accusation in her voice. She was absolutely correct; had her doctors simply taken a family history and offered her the BRCA testing at the time of her DCIS, she would have probably considered a risk-reducing (prophylactic) oophorectomy. This procedure only requires the removal of the tubes and the ovaries—anything else can be left intact. And if performed early, before ovarian cancer has started, the risk reduction by this surgery is over 90 percent. But most of all, for Victoria, it probably would have meant less surgery, no chemotherapy, and a much better prognosis. She still has to worry now that her tumor might come back.

We then talked about her risk for other cancers, including hers for more breast cancer and to develop pancreatic cancer. With trepidation I waited for her to ask me about my thoughts on whether she should go back and have a mastectomy, but was glad to talk about the elephant in the room when she finally did. She knew I was a strong proponent of BRCA testing and had a bilateral mastectomy myself despite evidence and risk factors to the contrary.

"Did you discuss the options with your breast surgeon initially and when you knew you had the mutation?" I asked her, trying to better understand her decision-making process at the time.

"Initially, the DCIS was located in one spot and a lumpectomy seemed to be the right thing, and I had radiation," she explained. "When I learned about the ovarian cancer diagnosis, I was just too overwhelmed with the surgery and chemotherapy, I just could not even think of having more surgery," she said, looking at me for reassurance.

"This is quite all right, for now," I said gently. "As long as you keep up with your mammograms and MRIs every year, and make sure you get a clinical exam."

Early on after a diagnosis of ovarian cancer, the risk of dying from ovarian cancer supersedes the risks of dying from a recurring breast cancer. An early recurrence from ovarian cancer carriers a very poor prognosis. With each passing year, that risk gets lower. With time her risk for more breast cancer will increase. And at some point, her risk for breast cancer would outweigh that for ovarian cancer and should prompt a further discussion about more breast surgery.

The discussion with Victoria, who is a well-connected scientist with perhaps more options than the average patient, once more brought home how important it for patients with BRCA mutations to receive care at a center with expertise, at least until the testing and the treatment for patients with BRCA mutations and their families becomes a routine part of medical care. Otherwise, these important connections between past and present may be overlooked—and cost much more in human lives and emotional toll than any out-of-pocket bill.

This is one of the main reasons that my colleagues and I

created our center for BRCA research: to provide a clinic and research center for men and women with hereditary cancer and BRCA mutation. We have the technology now to prevent ovarian cancer in women with BRCA mutation before it becomes incurable. A woman diagnosed with Stage I ovarian cancer has an over 90 percent chance to survive five years—but if she's diagnosed at Stage IV, this drops to 17 percent.

The last decade has brought many advances for patients like Madelaine, who, against all odds, lived nineteen years with her metastatic ovarian cancer.

For most of her treatment, Madelaine worked full-time and her side effects were tolerable. Being part of numerous clinical trials, she benefited from many of the newer treatments. Madeleine would come to clinic always upbeat and cheerful; and when her hair would fall out from the chemotherapy, she would wear one of those incredibly cute hats that one can only find in Paris. As is the case with many patients with a BRCA mutation, most of the chemotherapies she received worked better and much longer than they do in other patients with ovarian cancer without the mutation. Why is this? Cancer cells from patients with BRCA mutation are more vulnerable to drugs that affect DNA repair. Errors in cell replication happen constantly and are particularly common in cells, such as cells that are dividing. As part of the normal function, the BRCA genes help repair such defects. When the BRCA function is lost in a patient with BRCA mutation, it can no longer help repair DNA strand breaks. Thus when a patient receives chemotherapy that causes DNA strand breaks, tumor cells with faulty BRCA genes will not be able to protect themselves from the damage or repair it, whereas in cells with intact BRCA function, the tumor cells often actually find way to escape the effects of chemotherapy.

Great recent advances in the treatment for all BRCA cancers have come through clinical trials of ovarian cancer patients and the development of poly ADP ribose polymerase (PARP) inhibitors. While the BRCA mutation manages to turn healthy tissue into cancer, cancers with a BRCA mutation are very susceptible to chemotherapy and other agents that act by causing DNA breaks. For a long time, researchers have tried unsuccessfully to stamp out the BRCA mutation in the tumors. And then a very thoughtful group of researchers, including my coleader of the BRCA center for research at UCSF, Alan Ashworth, devised another strategy—and developed a group of new drugs that actually exploit the vulnerability of BRCA-mutated cancers. The first PARP inhibitor, olaparib, was approved for ovarian cancer in 2014, quickly followed by two other PARP inhibitors (niraparib, rucaparib) with likely more to come.

Being close to a research center, Madelaine was able to get in a clinical trial with a PARP inhibitor long before it was approved, as she did later with several similar drugs. For her the BRCA mutation gave her cancer, but it also gave her time. Because of these trials, she was able to raise her children and watch her son enter medical school—the two years he spent with us in the clinical trial unit got him hooked—six months before she died.

It is people like Madeline who help me answer how I can be an oncologist when it exposes me to so much sadness. It is for people like her that I spend so many extra hours in the laboratory to discover new treatment strategies and design new clinical trials.

Standing beside incredible women like Victoria and Madeline, who took their diagnoses in stride and utmost grace, also helped me go ahead with my risk-reducing oophorectomy within four short weeks of learning of my own mutation. Knowing full well how hard another surgery would be on my husband and my kids, I mentally accepted the surgery and I braced myself for going into menopause overnight. I couldn't give up yet, couldn't turn down my chance to be spared all of this simply because it had been a difficult year. I counted my blessings that I was lucky enough to have found out about my mutation in time.

Chapter 8

Prostate Cancer:
BRCA Mutations Don't Spare Men

O nce I made up my mind, I proceed with the oophorectomy in early December, less than four weeks after learning of my mutation. This surgery was relatively easy. Two days later, I learned I didn't have ovarian cancer and hoped this outcome meant my fateful year would have no more complications. A week later when my last stitches came out, I could not help but feeling a deep sense of accomplishment for pushing through all the surgeries in less than eight months. It had been a difficult year and I had done everything possible to reduce my risks of dying from cancer now and in the future. I knew at some level I would have to think of other cancers that come with this mutation, but for now the two most common cancers for my age were extinguished. And life could finally resume.

By spring, I truly felt I had adjusted. Work was as busy as ever—though now I was more mindful, succumbing to stress less often, and made a point to spend more time with the kids and exercise regularly (I may have been turning into Grandma a bit). Whenever sadness overwhelmed me, I would lace up my running shoes and jog along the water or up the hills. No matter how tired or grumpy I felt before I started, running would always bring back the peace of knowing how lucky I was to be here. Even today, when the moments of doubt inevitably arise, I am motivated to push on and advocate for more awareness about the BRCA mutation, which is still often thought of as only a mutation for breast and ovarian cancer even by people who should be in the know.

Late in spring of that year, I was invited to participate in a scientific panel to share my experience with BRCA as a patient and researcher. The first speaker from our four-member panel was a young woman who was diagnosed with breast cancer in her forties. She had presented with a large tumor that had gone undiagnosed for a while as no one, including herself, had thought she had breast cancer. She was later found to have a BRCA mutation and underwent chemotherapy and hormonal therapy. She told the audience that while she will likely survive the breast cancer, the chemotherapy, hormonal therapy, and removal of her ovaries had caused insufferable side effects. Stripped of all female hormones, she was physically and emotionally crippled such that she had not been able to go back to work even a year later. The audience was completely silent, mesmerized by her story. But I was not entirely sure whether the men and women in the room fully understood the extent of her suffering—and how much of this could have been prevented.

After her testimonial, two of the other panel members who were physicians shared their recent research advancements for

BRCA-related breast and ovarian cancer. Then it was my turn. Looking up, I could tell that the audience was watching me expectantly. Just by reading the brochure, it was clear that I was an expert in the disease and carrying its burden.

As the host began to introduce me and asked me to talk about my experience, a neatly dressed man in the audience got up, walked to the microphone, and asked to tell his story first. Gladly, I deferred to him, questioning now whether I really wanted to be up here telling my story and how I could bail. He introduced himself as Robert. He then explained that when he was in his early thirties, his mother had lost a long battle with ovarian cancer. She lived nearby and he had been with her through most of her treatments. Shortly before she died, his mother learned that she was a BRCA2 carrier.

"Everything is a bit of a blur now—it was a difficult time with Mom dying—but I clearly remember the agonizing weeks we waited for my sister's BRCA test to come back," he said softly into the microphone. His sister had just turned thirty-five and was about to get married. In those days, the test took four to six weeks to come back.

"I am sure you can imagine how happy we all were to find out that my sister did not have this gene. Mom was so relieved, she cried for hours at the news," he added.

"Yet, somehow, no physician or family adviser connected the dots. It was completely missed that I, myself, could also be a carrier of the BRCA mutation."

Through his mother he had a 50 percent chance of carrying the gene. Although he was a research scientist, the necessity for him to be tested for BRCA2 had never even crossed his mind, either. His mother's loss left such a void, he admitted that he just put the thought of the BRCA2 mutation in the family out of his mind and tried to move on.

Then two years ago just before he turned forty-five, he had a physical exam to apply for a life insurance policy. His doctor suggested that as part of the routine they check a PSA level, a marker for the detection of early-stage prostate cancer, with a simple blood test that can be done at pretty much any lab.

Robert told us that he had been a bit surprised by the doctor's recommendation. Like many health care professionals and the general public, he had closely followed the media controversy on PSA testing, an overall relatively inexpensive and painless screening. Just that year, some of the major American cancer and urological societies had started questioning in earnest whether the current practices for PSA testing were excessive and recommended against early and general PSA testing for men with an average risk for prostate cancer under the age of fifty-five. Since he was not African American (which would elevate his risk) and no one in his family had ever had prostate cancer, he considered himself average risk and safe for another ten years.

The reasons for the recommendations against the screening for men with average or low risk are similar to the discussions for breast cancer screening with mammograms. In average-risk men, the chance for the PSA blood test to be falsely elevated is much greater than the likelihood of finding cancer itself; a false positive test subjects more men to unnecessary prostate imaging and biopsy to either find no cancer or cancer that does not need treatment. Of course, these guidelines are not completely set in stone and many physicians may still order the test, often because they have a suspicion and sometimes "just to be on the safe side."

Robert suspected his own doctor fell in the wanting-to-be-safe camp, so he agreed without much questioning. That made it all the more surprising for both him and his doctor when his PSA came back very high. He also had the family's BRCA2 gene.

Here Robert paused in his story, choking up. When he found his voice again, he looked pleadingly at the panel: "What followed was a most horrendous year. I was diagnosed with a very aggressive form of prostate cancer. No one could tell me how long I have had it, but by the time I was diagnosed, the cancer had already spread to the lymph nodes outside the prostate. Fortunately, my surgeons were able to take the prostate and these lymph nodes out. To make sure that there were no tumor cells outside the surgical area, I got radiation afterward in the area where the prostate had been. I am now on hormonal therapy for another year. Had I only known that I carry the BRCA gene, I could have been screened years earlier and the cancer would probably have been found at an earlier stage. I wish I could have spared my wife this hardship."

He stopped talking and looked at us on the panel and then turned back to the audience. All of our eyes were moist hearing the testimony of this handsome man who at first appeared to be in the prime of his life. A woman in the audience stifled an audible sob. By the way he looked at her, it was clear she was his wife.

Desperately holding back my tears, I was glad to know that most of the people in the audience really were not fully aware of the enormity of his situation. And yet with much sadness, I realized this also meant most of the people in the room were not able to understand just how incredibly brave this man was to come forward with his story.

What Robert didn't explain was that together the prostatectomy and radiation therapy left him with a considerable chance of being impotent and incontinent for a long period, even permanently. And if he were lucky enough to have been spared these devastating side effects in the long run, for now the two years of hormonal therapy with an androgen blocker pill and monthly injections were completely shutting down his testosterone production. It has been known for many decades that testosterone itself fuels prostate cancer, so cutting off the testosterone supply in someone who has cancer can shrink a tumor and prevent it from spreading. An excess of testosterone can increase energy, drive, anger, and aggression, and decrease compassion, generosity, and empathy. Without it, some or all of these emotions can flip, depending on how strongly a man is controlled by his testosterone. During hormonal therapy, he is effectively castrated for the duration of the treatment, and perhaps a completely different person psychologically.

I thought I'd been through a lot having had fundamental organs of my womanhood removed. I should have been able to empathize, but as a woman I will never be able to really understand or describe what this must have felt like for Robert and others in his shoes. Testosterone is a driving force of everything male. Through the centuries, wars and quarrels have arisen from the excess of testosterone and most of the great stories of history probably would not have been written without the drive of this powerful male hormone. Admittedly, more than once I wished to see less of it from some of my male colleagues; any woman in science could tell you how big a role gender plays in our field.

For some men, a world can come apart with the loss of testosterone. A patient who had been treated with hormonal treatment for a period when he was forty, and in the midst of successful career as a venture capitalist, put it memorably: "Imagine you are racing in the America's Cup, hanging over the edge, straining against the wind, the spray of cold water in your face. In that moment you feel fully alive brimming with energy. And then all of a sudden the wind is gone from your sails. And just from yours. Any energy is gone from every fiber of your body. Not being able to be with my wife is just one of many things I have lost."

About 2.9 million men in the US are currently living with prostate cancer—it is the most common cancer in men. Fortunately, in the majority of these men, prostate cancer does not spread beyond the prostate gland, and as long as it is slow growing and does not invade surrounding organs like the bladder or other organs, prostate cancer does not require treatment. Most men are diagnosed with prostate cancer in later years of their lives, and very often men will die of other causes long before this cancer becomes fatal. In fact, in autopsy reports from men over eighty who died of other causes, almost 100 percent of them were found to have prostate cancer that most never knew they had in life. Until recently, many men with localized prostate cancer were offered prostatectomies or radiation to the prostate to prevent prostate cancer from becoming metastatic. However, the majority of men probably did not need such drastic measures. With the recognition that many prostate cancers don't require an intervention, a very large group of men with an increased PSA and a slow-growing tumor are undergoing "watchful waiting" without any form of active treatment. More recently the conservative approach to prostate cancer has been redefined as "active surveillance." It typically includes for these men to have a PSA test and a digital rectal exam every six months, and a prostate biopsy every one to two years. The majority of men will do just fine.

However, not everybody is so fortunate. About twenty-six thousand men each year in the US alone die from an aggressive form of prostate cancer, suggesting that an active intervention may be needed and is beneficial in a substantial number of men.

A man whose tumor becomes more aggressive will typically be offered either surgery to remove the prostate or radiation. Both procedures cause damage to the nerves and other tissues around the prostate and often are associated with a considerable risk for impotence and incontinence, and often with detrimental impact on quality of life. If the tumor shows signs of spreading, systemic hormonal therapy is added for six months to three years. Hormonal therapy with the goal to bring down testosterone to minimal levels—such as what Robert received—is only needed in cases of advanced prostate cancer, justifying efforts to detect prostate cancer early.

On the surface it seems like a policy of more and earlier screenings is the way to avoid the fates of these twenty-six thousand men. Since there is such a high cure rate of early-stage prostate cancer, much emphasis has been placed on early detection involving broad-population PSA screening, digital rectal exams, and MR imaging. However, the argument is not so clear cut. As we've seen, it is often not clear which prostate cancers are truly going to become aggressive and spread. And more so, not every man with prostate cancer will need treatment. Even metastatic tumors are often not aggressive enough to cause death. We just don't yet quite know in an individual man whether his particular tumor is deadly. A further complication in this debate is similar to one for breast and ovarian cancer: The removal of the prostate regardless of tumor malignancy does not work in every man, and often despite the surgery, the tumors become metastatic. The research on whether prostatectomies or prostate radiation truly can save lives is not consistent. Some reports suggested a clear benefit from radical prostatectomy versus watchful waiting; however, a recent study compared surgery, radiation, and active surveillance in over 1,600 men with prostate cancer diagnosed by routine PSA screening and found that the chance of dying from prostate cancer was not different for any three interventions. Nonetheless, for the men in the active surveillance group, many had tumors during the observation period that were advancing or spreading and ended up needing aggressive therapy and hormonal therapy over the course of the study. In fact, by ten years, 55 percent of the men randomized initially to active surveillance had required a radical intervention. The trauma of repeated biopsies and the anxieties associated with the frequent PSA tests during active surveillance may not be easy on every man and is fairly costly. The uncertainty and considerable risk for clinical progression and metastatic disease makes active surveillance a difficult choice for many men, in particular men of a young age with many years to worry. All in all these factors, as in other cancers, point to the strong need for better assessment of who is at risk and localized treatment options, with fewer and less severe side effects. Whether and in whom active surveillance is the best option will remain an ongoing struggle until we have a better understanding of who has a high risk. However, we know that among those with BRCA mutation, a man like Robert is at higher risk.

In a man with a BRCA mutation and elevated PSA, all this is very different. The mutation to look out for in men is the faulty BRCA2 gene, which is more readily linked to prostate cancer as opposed to BRCA1. (That said, even men with BRCA1 should be screened.) Whereas a mutated BRCA2 gene may cause fewer ovarian cancers and later breast cancer in women, mutations in this gene cause a far more aggressive form of prostate cancer, and the cancers occur at a much younger age. Carriers of a BRCA2 mutation are much less likely to survive their prostate cancer.

We used to think that BRCA mutations in prostate cancer were rare and only occurred in about 1 percent of all men with prostate cancer. However, more sophisticated testing showed that in men in whom the cancer has spread and become metastatic, over 10 percent of them carried a BRCA or similar mutation in the family, confirming that BRCA2 causes aggressive prostate cancers. Knowing about the mutation would not only help us in diagnosing prostate cancer at an earlier age, but it guides the therapy for those with advanced prostate cancer. As in women with ovarian cancer, PARP inhibitors have shown to be very effective for BRCA-related prostate cancer, offering these men a better tolerated and more effective option. PARP inhibitors are highly effective in killing cancers that have a defect in repairing DNA breaks, a hallmark of BRCA-related tumors. The introduction of these drugs for men with BRCA mutations has shown a real flash of hope of what otherwise often would be a fatal disease. On top of this, the emotional support and foresight men would gain by knowing their hereditary cancer should not be underestimated.

The same is true for men with BRCA-related male breast cancer, who often present late because they are not aware of their risk. If a man is aware of his risk to get breast cancer, finding it should be very easy. Often lumps can be felt when they are really small; mammograms pick up tumors easily in men. Early intervention will make it a highly curable disease, requiring only minimal surgery when diagnosed early. A prophylactic mastectomy in a man leaves very few traces when performed by an experience surgeon. Breast cancer in a man has a similar outcome as in a woman with the disease. Still, early diagnosis and recovery can be complex for men when they "enter a world of pink" and a waiting room full of women. One of my patients with male breast cancer, a successful lawyer, would beg me to sneak him into the mammogram suite through the back entrance so he did not have to feel like an intruder and suffer the curious or even hostile glances of all the women sitting in the mammography waiting room. No amount of reassurance made him feel any less out of place. And even with support of friends and family, he admitted that he did not feel comfortable discussing his experiences with friends and colleagues or even admit that he had breast cancer. Eliminating the emotional taboos of male breast cancer would allow an early diagnosis and an extremely good outcome. With the increasing BRCA testing in men, and an active screening effort, it is time to recognize the immense impact that emotional support and resources will have for a man with breast cancer, and any man with a BRCA mutation should have easy access to medical programs centered on hereditary cancer. No man should die of breast cancer because he felt too embarrassed to have a mammogram.

Had Robert known that he carried the mutation, his prostate cancer may not have been prevented, but it would have been likely found at an earlier stage, requiring less surgery and no radiation and hormonal therapy. He would have had his PSA checked from the time when he turned forty and would have been examined regularly at least once a year, if not more often. Hopefully in the near future, a clinical trial with newer strategies to prevent prostate cancer altogether will be developed. This is what Robert pleaded for—for men from families with known BRCA mutations get tested to be spared his fate.

And hopefully we will get there soon so by the time my sons reach their thirties, we will have more sophisticated tests and targeted therapies for BRCA-related cancers so they are spared my fate.

I had been asked to sit on that panel to talk about my experience as a patient and my research, but more than anything I wanted to talk about my hopes and obligations to twist all our fates and make life safer for patients with BRCA mutations. Inspired, I went to my clinic, confident that my trepidation about whether I could continue as an oncologist were easing away. I began to accept that I was a doctor and a patient.

Chapter 9

Back to Normal:
Feeling, and Fighting, the Cancer Blues

"Your exam looks fine; I cannot find any evidence of your tumor in the skin or lymph nodes. Your lungs are clear and everything else looks normal to me." I couldn't have been more excited to give such good news to a patient like Lis, who was well into the second year of her diagnosis of metastatic breast cancer. She would see me every month in clinic and she was doing well over the last two years. We were the same age and both had three kids, and over the last months had grown very close as we talked about our families and matters beyond breast cancer during her visits. Thinking my evaluation was a high enough note to end on, I walked over to the sink to wash my hands and get ready to go. But before I could turn on the faucet she stopped me: "Do you think this is a good time to exchange my implants?"

I must have shot her my "Where did that come from?" look. I knew she had had reconstruction more than ten years earlier, after her first diagnosis, so it had been a while. But medically the implants were safe with very little tissue reaction, and cosmetically her reconstruction looked fine.

She paused. "Please don't think that I am vain, but I think I am ready to change my implants and improve a few things here and there. If there are any advances in the techniques and new options for implants, I would like to discuss them.

"Don't get me wrong." An apologetic smile crossed her face, as if she was for a moment uncertain whether to go on. "I am totally content and have gotten used to the reconstructions, the scars, and the looks. I really like my cosmetic result, and I am quite aware that not everybody is as lucky as I've been.

It had only been about seven months since my own surgery and I felt myself tense while listening to her. Having taken care of many patients who had undergone either a one-sided or bilateral mastectomy, I knew that the majority of women always remain somewhat sad to have lost their breasts. However, regardless of whether the surgery was done by choice or by necessity, very few women ultimately regretted the decision of having a mastectomy. Having peace of mind of being definitively cancer-free counts for a great deal. As I looked at Lis now, I saw the courageous young woman who had undergone a double mastectomy "to leave no stone unturned"; and even after having metastatic disease anyway, she did not seem to regret her decision. Standing next to her by the examining table, I felt a sudden feeling, a pang of angst. I knew that mastectomies really don't save lives in the majority of women, and what if I had done this extensive surgery in vain? It still felt all so very raw for me.

"How long did it take you to come to terms with losing your breasts?" I blurted out, instinctively crossing my arms in front of my chest.

Clearly surprised by my question, she did not reply immediately. I averted my gaze, forgetting for a moment that I was the physician in this relationship. I could feel her eyes scrutinizing my chest. When she looked back up, she had a knowing impression in her eyes.

"Why are you asking?" She searched my face for answers.

At that time, I was still uneasy about talking to patients about my own breast cancer—let alone mentioning it during clinic visits. It was too vulnerable a confession, and since I was still uncertain of what patients would think of a physician going through a similar process as theirs, I really did not think I should take precious time from their visits. Would they consider me less able to do my job if they knew I'd been sick, that I hadn't been able to save myself from the disease I treated every day?

Lis, however, was different. I knew I had a special bond with her, and in this particular moment I was torn between needing encouragement from someone who had gone through my present struggles, and needing to toe the line between professional and personal relationships. Focusing on the medical chart in front of me, I remained silent for a long moment and hoped she might forget my question.

When I realized her inquiring eyes weren't leaving me, I took a deep breath and responded. "I had a double mastectomy six months ago, and I wonder how one copes with it in the end."

"How are you feeling?" she asked me. She quietly reached out for my hand.

I slowly pondered the question, and then realized that I really was not quite ready to talk about it.

"Well, given the circumstances," I deflected and then launched into an extended explanation, to answer her question, about the latest advances in breast reconstruction. Talking doctorly about medicine, in technicalities and jargon, brought me back into my comfort zone.

Sensing how torn I felt, she didn't delve deeper. Instead we talked more about possible options for her to revise her reconstruction.

"Do you think it is worth it for me, and do you have any medical concerns?"

Unspoken in her question were the ultimate questions—first, whether I thought she would live long enough for the surgery to make sense; and second, the fear that because she had metastatic breast cancer, it would be difficult to find a surgeon to agree to another extensive surgery just for "cosmetic" reasons. Her concerns were quite justified, because more often than not, I had been told by a colleague that such a surgery would not make sense if the person were going to die in the next couple of months or years.

"I think you look beautiful," I said, "but you had saline implants. There are newer implants that look and feel nicer and you would be much happier with. Most of them are now silicone-based, and after extensive testing for more than a decade, they've now been deemed safe. The initial concerns about leaking have been resolved, and their shape and consistency has improved over saline. There are still some worries with a subtype of implants that have been linked to an unusual type of lymphoma, but they are exceedingly rare, and I don't think our surgeons use these types anyway."

Then, looking directly into her eyes and holding her gaze, I added, "I have no hesitation for you to go through a revision from an oncology standpoint. With your permission, I will refer you to a wonderful plastic surgeon who is both technically very good and who will be very sensitive to your questions and special circumstances."

As her visit drew to a close, she gave me another encouraging look, an opening to talk about myself now that her turn was over. I could not quite understand why, but at the time I felt so out of sorts and knew I was not yet ready to talk. At least not with Lis. How could I be upset about my situation, when Lis's diagnosis had this vastly different dimension? How could I have put this burden on my patient, to doctor her doctor? My DCIS was a thing of the past, while she would have to deal with metastatic breast cancer for the rest of her life. I regretted losing control for that moment and showing the side of myself I normally keep closed up inside my white coat.

I started toward the door, ready and eager to move onto the next patient, when I heard Lis say quietly, "I am happy to talk, when you're ready. Just because my diagnosis may be worse than yours, it doesn't mean you are not allowed to struggle with yours. You have been such a rock in my care, I would love being of some help to you. Please reach out anytime."

I nodded and gave her a hug. "Thank you, and I truly appreciate your offer, but here at the clinic, the focus is all about you."

With a forced smile, I left the examination room. Needing a short reprieve before seeing my next patient, I stepped out into the stairwell and sat on the steps.

How *did* I feel? I really didn't know how to answer this.

On one hand, I felt really lucky. I only had Stage 0 breast cancer, and other than having bruises and scars, I would be fine—there was very little real threat to my life even in the long run. My chance of survival should be close to 100 percent. My reconstruction surgeries were also completed without any complication, and I had virtually no physical compromise. So, should I then not be well on the way to feeling better? I had had many sports-related surgeries in my life, and I remember the pain being less of a frustration than the physical limitations during recovery. Life went on even after I was cut open. So, why was this so different?

It's true that for most patients, the physical recovery appears much quicker than the emotional recovery. After the initial hectic pandemonium of decision-making, all energies are geared toward getting through treatment, dealing with side effects, and holding your life together. The mechanics of therapy in early-stage breast cancer or any other curable cancer are fairly straightforward. Surgery, chemotherapy, radiation therapy, in this order, or variations of it. Lots of support from family and friends—frequent and reassuring visits with the medical team. A clearly structured, and mostly well-supported, blueprint to fight for life. I was an intensely busy professional with little wiggle room in my life for anything. Fitting cancer into my hectic work and parenting schedule had really not been that easy; but somehow, I'd managed to get through it. Now, all of that was over—life should have gone back to normal. Somehow, it just had not.

The previous day, as I walked the hall to my office, I looked at the ever so familiar names of my colleagues on their office doors: "Dr. Bergsland," "Dr. Warren," "Dr. Jahan." As a patient, I no longer felt a part of this group of doctors, my colleagues. But now that I was back in clinic seeing patients with real problems, I did not feel I belonged here as a patient anymore, either. In fact, I almost felt ashamed that I was not happy—ungrateful that I could not appreciate having been so fortunate.

What I had previously only witnessed from observing patients, I was now experiencing. In the middle of a very busy clinic, I was suddenly gripped by fears that I could not articulate. I would see a patient who only had DCIS and yet her tumor had spread to the liver—and my confidence that I would be fine completely vanished. Would this be me?

I had lost my identity. I was stuck in between my old "medically carefree" self and this new state that I could not yet define. I had lost my sense of immortality, my optimism for the resilience of life.

One night, I dreamed I received a phone call that the tumors had spread to my brain. Disoriented and panicked, I woke up and fumbled for my phone in the dark; it was indeed ringing, but it was a doctor from the emergency room calling me about a mutual patient. Thoughts of brain tumors had become my literal nightmare that caught me completely off guard. I could read an obituary of someone who died at age eighty-five, and fall into a bottomless pit thinking I would never get to that age.

All that I was experiencing was all too familiar to me. I had heard it many times, in text books, blogs, and countless conversations with patients in my clinic. Patients had told me that they could not stop crying for days, or had sudden crying spells, unprovoked and unpredictable. Common to most testimonies was that no amount of reassurance that the prognosis was excellent, or the steadfast support of family and friends would help. Often patients even actually did not want to impose on family and friends more than they already had. The loneliness that a cancer diagnosis brings amid so many well-wishers is difficult to explain. For many patients, this period, for which I am still striving to find a good name—feels similar to a car crash that one survives. The visuals remain long after the bruises have healed. Physically the worst was over. I had done everything above and beyond what was needed to survive this cancer. The imminent danger had dissipated, and yet unlike the physical events, my emotions had not been resolved and deep down, my mind was stuck in the fears and threats, while outwardly everything seemed fine.

This does not just happen for those patients with a diagnosis of cancer. I'm reminded of one of my young patients who had had a risk-reducing bilateral mastectomy and oophorectomy for a BRCA1 mutation to prevent cancer. She came through the surgeries with flying colors. At the visit just after completing her surgery and reconstruction, she beamed at me and enthusiastically told me that she now had everything behind her, and she was ready to take on any battle that lie ahead. She tried to convince me so thoroughly that her life was great, and she could not wait to go back to her weight lifting and social life. Listening to her, I was not entirely certain whether she was trying to convince me that she was fine, or herself. And maybe, I hoped she would be just fine.

"I am glad you're through all of your surgeries, and it is wonderful to see how well you are doing," I said reassuringly. "However, it's not uncommon that in the next few months, the reality of losing your breast and going into early menopause will make you sad. It may take a good twelve to eighteen months to recover and find your bearings again. Please know that I am always here for you." She looked at me, not really understanding what I was trying to say. I felt a twinge of remorse for spoiling her high. A year later, though, she told me how true my words had been. In later conversations she shared that it took her almost two years to put the surgeries behind her, and as an afterthought, how glad she was that she knew that it would take time.

Sitting in that stairwell, I should have been saying all of these words to myself. The "cancer blues" can span a very broad range from difficulty coping with the new situation to a reactivation of post-traumatic stress for those with known trauma in their past, or even to overt depression. For some, it may just be survival jitters; these feelings can span a very broad range.

My self-imposed pressure to feel constantly happy—to have survived cancer—really wreaked havoc with my emotions. As a doctor, I usually feel upbeat, finding ways to encourage patients and be optimistic. I had many of those days, profoundly grateful to be well healed and ready to move on. But then there were the days when I *just wasn't feeling it*. Once, when I was completely frustrated trying to meet another deadline, one of my colleagues said somewhat jokingly to me, "You know, you are just human; you could give yourself a little bit of a break." I bristled at her. Being out of control was not who I was. She smiled caringly at me and told me to "be kind to myself" and accept that healing and restoring a healthy sense of femininity after any type of breast surgery takes time. For some reason *being kind to myself* stuck more than *giving myself a break*; reminding myself of that phrase became one of those very simple tricks that was actually very helpful in accepting my new situation.

As a researcher and clinician, I knew that within two to three years, almost everyone is back to where they started before the diagnosis. I could anticipate it and prepare them for it, but lacking the technical language and procedures and treatments I relied on for healing the physical side effects of treatment, I wasn't always equipped with the remedies it takes to help emotional recovery. Now, I know that just understanding what someone goes through is its own kind of medicine.

Why go through the process of surgery if it's so emotionally and physically fraught? Restoring the breasts after mastectomy, either with an implant or natural tissue, or even correction of a disfiguring lumpectomy, is not at all a vain process. It's actually an integral part of healing and recovery. Women who undergo breast reconstruction are much less likely to get depressed and in general are more content in the long run. Good surgical outcomes are always important, but in this case seem a bit more so to solidifying the patient's sense of self. It's worth it to make the final result as flawless as possible—even if it means taking an extra step.

It's an unkind myth that surgical reconstruction does not matter in older women, particularly in a disease that is so much more common in older women. No doctor should really just accept when a woman starts with the question, "Why at my age should I . . . ?" No one is ever too old for reconstruction. Even if older women initially may think good cosmetics are no longer important, it is quite clear that the emotional health and recovery are much better for those who undergo reconstruction. Several studies show that there should be no age limit to offer reconstruction, and there is also very little evidence that older women have more complications. There are many reports, both scientific and in the lay press, comparing the satisfaction of one type of procedure versus the other. For every woman, the choice of the appropriate surgery should be based on an in-depth discussion with her surgery team; and it is quite okay to seek a second opinion, or to ask whether the surgeon can actually perform all the options that are feasible. The conversation can be difficult and feel too personal, so it may be helpful to bring a friend along who can ask the important questions. In the end, it is your body. Regrets usually are linked to having been poorly informed and not understanding risks; however, no one should ever feel forced to have reconstruction, as it may well be that a woman may not want to proceed after hearing all the options for reconstruction. Nonetheless, choosing among options is always preferred to feeling like there is only one fate. And reconstruction can be done at any time later.

For some women, at least in the short term, the cancer blues may turn into depression and may need to be treated with antidepressants. Symptoms of prolonged feelings of depression, the inability to find pleasure in daily life, or losing interest in familiar activities should prompt further evaluation for major depression, and may eventually hamper cancer recovery. The degree of depression has very little to do with the magnitude of the illness and can be exacerbated by lingering effects of chemotherapy, or in those who poorly tolerate hormonal therapy. In fact, in one of our early studies, we learned that coping with cancer therapy may be worse in those with Stage 0 and I disease. For those who struggled with depression before the cancer, or who have had significant trauma in the past, a cancer diagnosis may bring back past depression and trauma. Depression is actually exceedingly common also absent of the diagnosis of cancer. Depression can interfere with sleep, eating, energy, concentration, and self-image—or even cause recurrent thoughts of death or suicide. Even if it is difficult for you to reach out during a low period or if you may need an intervention, it is important to know that things will get better.

It's clear by now that cancer can strain a patient's relationship with herself, but it can also completely shift and upset any outside relationship. Many caregivers (male and female) are at sea or overwhelmed by the ever-changing and often demanding needs of a cancer patient. I have seen the most supportive marriages and friendships come apart; but I've also seen love flourish completely unexpectedly. I still remember with profound gratitude, how cared for I felt during all my surgeries. But sometimes cancer just becomes too overwhelming, and the most endearing relationship does not survive.

Like most people, I thought I was pretty astute when it came to human relationships; but about five years ago, I was completely blindsided by Riley, a very young patient with met-astatic breast cancer, and her caring husband, Chad. On their first visit, Chad was almost overbearing in advocating for Riley's care. He would spare no cost; only the best treatment would do for his beloved wife. He politely pushed me to back up every treatment suggestion with precise evidence and tailored reasons for why I would choose it above any other options. Riley is so lucky to have the love and support of this caring man, I thought.

Six months later, her cancer stopped responding to the hor-monal therapy she was on, and she had more pain and difficulty sleeping. Her scans showed worsening, so I put her on a different therapy, once again under much scrutiny from Chad. But on her next appointment she was alone; when I asked where Chad was, she said, "Oh, he had a big project at work." The next month, no Chad and another quick excuse. At the fourth appointment, she told me that they were getting a divorce—she had already left their house and moved in with her sister. By extension, she was losing her insurance. Within a year, Chad and Riley would offi-cially part ways. When Riley told me all this, I at first had very cruel thoughts about Chad's behavior.

Until about eighteen months into Riley's treatment, when I was standing on line at the coffee shop near the hospital. The man behind me stepped closer to me and said hello. It was Chad—and all those negative thoughts came pouring into my heart like a flood. Not able to hide by anger, I acknowledged him with a deliberately reserved and rather icy tone. I had had a busy day and this short coffee break was the first moment I'd had for myself and he was the last person I wanted to spend that precious time with.

He looked at me, quickly realizing I was not in the mood for small talk.

"You know, I did not want this divorce," he said without preamble. I was unconvinced, and yet as I stared into his face, I noticed that he had very kind eyes. Eyes that were pleading with me to believe him.

With a sigh, I relented. "Would you like to talk about it? I have a few minutes," I offered, irritated that I let myself get pulled into a conversation with him in the first place. I grabbed my coffee, which no longer seemed so enticing, and sat down at one of the empty tables in the corner. He joined me, uncertain how to begin. I raised my eyebrows and glanced at my watch.

"I know you must think I'm a complete jerk," he began. "And you are right; I could have done so much better. I just didn't know how. She was just so sad all the time, and nothing I did was ever enough. I would try to be funny, and she'd burst into tears. I would try to hold her, and she would freeze up or push me away. I felt utterly helpless. And then I blew it."

The remorse in his voice dissolved my anger.

"It is too late for us now, but I really hope she will be okay," he added. "How is she?"

"You know I cannot talk about her with you, but I hope you can reach out to her, and tell her how you feel. Whether or not it is too late for your marriage, is not for me to judge. However, I am certain, she would appreciate your friendship." I stood up and offered my hand. "Thank you for sharing this me with me."

"Will you tell her?" he asked me.

"No, but I truly think you should."

As I walked back to the hospital, I could not help but feeling terribly remorseful. I should have checked in on Riley's emotional well-being so much more. Three years into her diagnosis, a new young man began coming with her to the visits. He introduced himself as Matt, "a friend." Matt joined her for a total of three visits, and his first absence reminded me of what had happened with Chad. Worried about her, I carefully asked where Matt was today.

"He's outside in the waiting room," she answered.

"Ah, you don't want him to come back here with you?"

"No, I wanted to do this alone today," she said with a hint of prickliness in her voice.

She was referring to our review of her recent scans and the discussion of whether her treatment was still working. It was a scheduled scan of her lungs and liver, as well as her spine and bones, which she usually had about every ten to twelve weeks.

"Are you sure? I am happy to have one of my staff members go out and get him," I offered. She shook her head.

I pulled up the images of her CT scans on the computer and showed her that all the tumors in the liver were shrinking. Clearly this chemotherapy was working. She also tolerated it fairly well—that day, I noticed how pretty she looked, and the hair she'd lost months ago was just starting to regrow.

"This is really good news, I am so glad you are doing well." And as I stood, she burst out in tears.

"Okay, so now that the good news is out of the way, let's talk about what's upsetting you—and why that gorgeous and caring man is sitting by himself in the waiting area," I said softly with a smirk, sitting down again.

"He is so nice and kind, but he deserves to be with some who is not going to die on him and who is not sick all the time." She sobbed, tearing streaming down her cheeks. Chad's words about how much she had pushed him away came back to me.

"Maybe," I replied. "But the fact is he is out there waiting for *you* and not someone else."

She pushed back. "I can't bear doing this to him. I'm going to die, and he'll have to watch."

Now with tears in my own eyes, I said, "Matt knows this. Don't push him away. Promise me that you will at least think about it." I hugged her tight and let her cry in my arms.

Over the next year, Matt taught Riley to surf. When she got weaker from her cancer and the effects of chemotherapy, he took her to Maui so she could sit on a terrace to watch the sunset. She died a year later with Matt at her side. She had just turned thirty-two. I still have the note from him thanking me for a most precious year in his life.

Thinking of Riley during my low phases, I reflected on what would help, how I could signal other people that I wanted and needed help. From afar she had willed me to reach out, even though it was very hard. Nevertheless, I was someone used to being in charge and in control, rarely really needing to reach out. As a physician, I had been trained to have difficult conversations. As a patient, I became aware how difficult it was for many people, even close friends, to approach the topic of cancer. More than one patient told me with bitterness that being told "You can beat this!" was really unhelpful and made her feel even more isolated than knowing she had an incurable disease and was likely going to die. I had to remind myself and my patients that most people don't have a lot of practice with difficult conversations about cancer, and some things just feel unbearable to talk about candidly. So steering the conversation toward a simple question—such as "How do you feel?" or "Do you want to talk about it?"—can go a long way, rather than allowing awkwardness to be mistaken for a lack of compassion. Or more concrete, "What can I do to help?" And as a patient, a small statement like "It is okay to talk about it!" often helps friends and family at a loss for words to start a conversation.

For me, much healing came from simple interventions and time. I remembered to be kind to myself over and over and in new ways. Exercise and sufficient sleep—a hard commodity to come by in my profession—became crucial. And both have solid data supporting their efficacy for cancer patients.

I always was fond of exercise, but when I was recovering, running became my safe space. Like my oversized labradoodle, Sampson, who will automatically start wagging his tail when I start tying my running shoes, running shot a ray of sunshine through any sadness I was feeling, and despite the real weather outside. The sound of my feet pounding the ground, my lungs on fire, my mind quieting—the perfect soundtrack for a worry-free hour.

At first glance, exercise may not be the solution for everyone. It may not have been part of a patient's life prior to cancer, or it may just simply tire them out too much even thinking about it. When you are feeling queasy and wiped out from chemotherapy, when all your joints hurt from hormonal therapy, when you're going through early menopause, or when you're yanked off estrogen replacement therapy, the last thing on your mind would be hitting the gym. Used as a collective term for several symptoms, *medical fatigue* includes not having any energy, feeling tired all the time, and feeling exhausted. Moreover, it is not linked to any particular activity, such as doing chores all day, working out, or other exertion. Usually, this fatigue is not relieved by resting, and the lack of energy can linger on for days or even weeks. Often patient and doctors alike are looking for drugs to help with fatigue—wouldn't it be great to just be able to take a pill and feel better?

Fatigue can be particularly troublesome. Ironically, however, the thing people avoid because of fatigue is exactly what helps most. Exercise works wonders for our bodies on many levels, from reducing weight gain to improved cardiac health. Many studies even compared the benefits of exercise and psychological and drug interventions, and now there are results from data that have been collected from over ten thousand men and women who were randomly assigned to get a drug to combat fatigue, emotional support, or exercise. To the surprise of many, exercise decreased the cancer-related fatigue the most. And it didn't matter what type of exercise was practiced. It could be strenuous aerobic, such as running; anaerobic, such as lifting weights; or simply just walking. Most important, we learned from this study that such drugs as Provigil or Ritalin actually just don't work as well as exercise.

The point is all about finding solace, which is different for everybody. Just going outside and being immersed in nature may bring some reprieve for most patients. You may not be able to run, but surely there must a form of exercise that will work.

Chapter 10

Curse or Cure?
My Dad's BRCA-Related Pancreatic Cancer Story

I t was early summer again and the end of my roller-coaster year with breast cancer. I was back in control—past the diagnosis, the double mastectomy, reconstructive surgeries, removal of my ovaries, and frequent bouts of depression and fear. For the first few months after my diagnosis, I would look at all the faces of patients who were not doing well, and my only thought was that I could be one of them. Even on days when I was completely upbeat and confident that this was all behind me, anything could trigger a thought that the next cancer was lurking around the corner. But now, it was a year after my diagnosis; I'd just turned forty-nine and was training to run the Boston Marathon, besides coping with everyday life again. Slowly my confidence that I would be fine had come back, the thought of cancer receding. I had just come back from a business trip from China when my dad sent me the results of his recent abdominal ultrasound. Reading the email he sent, I instinctively knew that the BRCA gene had sprung out of our family closet once again.

A couple of weeks earlier, during one of our weekly Skype calls, my father mentioned that he was having a bit of stomach trouble. Healthy all his life and with no reason to worry about what seemed to be indigestion, he did not think much of it. He was seventy-eight, stoic by nature and very fit. He did not smoke and drank very little alcohol. Nonetheless, his doctor, a veteran in gastroenterology who has taken care of my dad for two decades, wanted to check it out.

In most men my father's age, digestive issues are common and have lots of causes that would not cause me to panic. But I did not think of ulcers or bad constipation when he mentioned having "a bit of stomach upset." My mind went directly to pancreatic cancer.

After I learned that I had the BRCA gene, we needed to figure out which parent had passed on the gene to me. On my mother's side, several family members had had colon cancer; but there was no breast or ovarian cancer. My mother herself was well in her seventies with no cancer and none in her family, so it's much less likely that she would be carrying the BRCA gene.

It had to be my father. On his side, also there were not many women with cancer, but there were only very few family members. He was a single child and his father died when he was thirty-six during the Second World War, as did his grandparents. His mother *did have* breast cancer; however, she was sixty-five when she was diagnosed, and one barely spoke about her diagnosis. Really, not a very typical story for a BRCA mutation. However, as we are learning now, there are many families with hereditary cancers like mine—untold stories of mutations that have gone undetected. And in hindsight, his maternal grandmother *had* died at twenty-nine, and of symptoms that could be explained by ovarian cancer.

In January 2013, genetic line testing only was offered to those with at least one family member with breast or ovarian cancer under the age of fifty and another young first-degree relative (parent, sibling, or child). Testing was also performed in those with family members carrying a BRCA mutation. He was tested and it soon became clear that my father carried the BRCA gene. And now less than five months later, here he was with abdominal pain. Fortunately for him, we knew that he carried the BRCA gene—and hence a higher risk for pancreatic and prostate cancer. At the time of his diagnosis, there were no recommendations to screen someone with a BRCA2 mutation for pancreatic cancer—and even today, such screening only occurs at large centers and among those who already know they carry the gene.

With very good reason, pancreatic cancer is much feared; and little has changed since I saw my first cases in medical school two decades ago. It is one of the deadliest cancers we know, partly because early detection rarely happens. About 53,000 men and women present each year with pancreatic cancer; and in spite of medical advances everywhere else, 43,000 people will die from it each year. Only about 5,000 of these patients present at an early stage where surgery is still an option. Even in these patients, the best of cases, surgery often comes too late and only 1 in 3 will survive five years beyond diagnosis. For most people who don't drink excessively or smoke, the risk for pancreatic cancer is about 1 percent over a lifetime and usually it happens later in life, most often in people's seventies. Women have slightly lower risk than men to develop pancreatic cancer, but not by much. The likelihood of surviving a year with advanced pancreatic cancer is less than 50 percent. Fewer than 10 percent survive five years and only the very lucky who are diagnosed at a very early stage will be among the long-term survivors. It was only eight months from the time my grandmother presented with her second cancer to her death.

For someone with a BRCA2 mutation, the risk for pancreatic is considerably higher and it occurs earlier than usual: in their late fifties and early sixties. Pancreatic cancer is the third most common cancer with BRCA mutation for both men and women, and many women with BRCA2-related pancreatic cancer already have had breast cancer. Those with other family members with pancreatic cancer should be aware that pancreatic cancer does run in families.

Sitting at my sunny kitchen table that morning in July 2013, with the abdominal ultrasound report in front of me, my heart sank. It showed a shadow in the area of the pancreas—not necessarily cancer, but still a shadow—so the gastroenterologist recommended that Dad have a further workup.

I spoke to his doctor, who tried reassuring me "that this is likely nothing to worry about." Just to be complete and because my father had a BRCA2 mutation, we agreed on getting a better look with a CT scan.

It took a few days to get the results back. They showed another lesion on his liver and a large mass either in or near his pancreas, but it was not clear what this mass was and whether it was a cancer. Tumors in the pancreas are notoriously difficult to clearly differentiate from other changes that are not cancerous, even by CT scan. This makes it very challenging for even a seasoned radiologist to be specific. Hence, the CT scan report gave us more information, but not anything useful. This is why experts now recommended an MRI for suspected pancreatic cancer.

By now, my father—an engineer who spent his life making precise and definitive measurements—was getting frustrated by the fact that, after two trips to the hospital for different imaging studies, he still had no definitive diagnosis. All we knew was that inside his body was a "large mass of uncertain etiology, worrisome for malignancy," and his doctors, he felt, bore a "fairly noncommittal attitude" about the whole thing. Unfortunately, this situation happens all too frequently. Unless a tumor in the pancreas is very advanced, the workup for pancreatic cancer is tedious and not very straightforward. Many patients, like my dad, go through multiple scans and biopsies that are inconclusive and the reports that are rather vague. One day after his last doctor's visit, he pointed out that if engineers built bridges the way "you," meaning doctors in general, practice medicine, a lot of people would be left hanging in the air. Of course, from the doctors' perspective, as long as there is nothing definitive pointing to cancer, we don't worry. Yet I know now that coming from the patients' perspective, only the *certainty* that this is *not* cancer is reassuring.

I tried to explain to him that CT scans are very good in searching for tumors but that once a tumor is suspected, a dedicated

MRI of a special organ is better at honing in on details. The next test—always the next test—would be more definitive.

Since this specific MRI requires special equipment and an expert in reading the images, he had to travel to a different town. When he got there, the nurse asked him to remove anything that contained metal and could be magnetic. She gave him a set of headphones to listen to music; he was placed on a movable table and then moved into a large, closed machine.

Compared to CT scans and X-rays, MRIs involve no radiation; however, being enclosed in something that looks like a sarcophagus, and the infernal banging from the vibration of the magnetic coils during the test, pushes many already anxious patients completely over the edge. MRIs must by absolutely frightening for someone like my dad who, as a child, spent many nights huddled in dark bomb shelters during World War II air raids.

Two more endless days passed before the report came back. This time there was nothing vague about it: Right there, clear as day, was a very large pancreas mass encroaching on his small bowel and wrapping itself around some of the blood vessels, definitely making this a bad cancer that could not be removed.

After this, things happened very fast. He was called back and underwent an endoscopic retrograde cholangio pancreatogram (ERCP) to take a piece of the tumor. After he received a mild sedative, a tube with camera was inserted through his mouth, passed through the esophagus, the stomach, and then backward through the bile duct into the pancreas. A piece of tissue was then extracted with a needle.

This procedure ended the mysterious battery of tests. The results were not good: pancreatic cancer. Despite his acting on his first symptoms and taking immediate action, and despite the precaution of his doctor and myself (the extra-protective doctor-relative), my father's tumor was advanced and could not be surgically removed. After finally having a diagnosis, we met with Dr. Schmied at the municipal hospital in St. Gallen. A man of imposing size and stature, he was an expert in pancreatic surgery, performing more than fifty such surgeries per year. He was kind, but no-nonsense. He walked us through all the images from the CT and MRI pictures, pointing out the size of the tumor and its invasion into the duodenum. Although he dismissed the surgical option, he was not trying to dismiss us, and he was very thorough in going through all the reasons that he was hesitant to perform surgery. Removing pancreatic cancers is very challenging, no matter what stage—such surgeries are only done by experienced surgeons. The process involves removing most or all of the pancreas, part of the small intestine, the gallbladder, parts of the bile duct, blood vessels, and surrounding lymph nodes. Besides the tedious work the surgeon must do, the patient suffers even more. Three to 4 percent don't survive the procedure, and those who do take months to recover, often have later complications, and need lifelong support with pancreatic enzymes and insulin. This is why the surgery is performed on only those who have a good chance of having all their tumors removed completely

Other treatments have a similarly low success rate. Most of the time, pancreatic cancer does not respond as well to chemotherapy as do other tumors; and if responsive at all, it takes three types of chemotherapy to shrink such tumors. These three chemotherapies are grueling on the body, often leaving the sturdiest of patients with profound side effects and weakness. Even if the chemo works, the tumor comes right back when the therapy is stopped; so many patients never really get a break from the chemotherapy.

Dr. Schmied explained to us all the reasons that surgery wasn't an option: Both my father's age and the advanced nature of the tumor made it a very dangerous—and most likely futile—endeavor. Furthermore, my dad's case had been presented at the hospital's tumor board, a meeting where many doctors (oncologists, surgeons, radiologists, pathologists) weigh in on a case, and everybody had agreed this surgery should not be attempted. Plus, would he want to spend the last years of his life in a prolonged and complicated recovery?

I know I failed as a daughter at that moment, because I barely heard anything Dr. Schmied said. Instead of diligently being the note-taker, the processor, of this information, I was entertaining vivid memories of many patients with whom Dr. Schmied had had this same conversation. Unfortunately, only those patients with a pancreatic tumor that can be removed completely have a reasonable chance of survival. However, most patients present at an unresectable stage, when the tumor can no longer be cut out.

I asked Dr. Schmied whether he would reconsider if we got Dad's tumor to shrink. I pointed out the special circumstances of the BRCA mutation and my dad's supreme fitness; even at his age, he bikes twenty miles on most days and hikes up the Swiss mountains on others. The chances that he'd recover well were surely higher as a result. As Dr. Schmied paused, I could tell he was debating whether to answer the daughter of his Swiss patient or the cancer expert from California. At this visit, as at all the others, my father's doctor looked past him, speaking only to me. Finally, Dr. Schmied said this would be highly unlikely. But that in principle, yes, if I thought of a way to make this happen, he would reconsider. He wished us all the best and left the room.

My father beamed in amazement. "Wow, you really are somebody!"

For my father, a stoic man, that was quite an admission. A realist who'd spent his youth in Hitler's Germany and lost his father and all his uncles to the war, the term *warm and fuzzy* does not exactly come to mind.

It was the beginning of an entirely new relationship. One that I know helped me push him to not give up during the difficult cancer journey ahead. There are few instances in life when you can truly apply your knowledge to save someone so close.

We drove back in silence, each of us deep in thought, sober. When we got home, Dad went into his garden, while Marietta and I made dinner, both of us desperately trying to hold it together. The conversation stayed light—and then, we went to bed.

The next morning, I woke up to a stunningly beautiful Swiss summer day. Dad and Marietta sat in the garden, and I joined them with a cup of coffee. My father looked at me with his deep blue eyes—even deeper that day. Like the BRCA mutation, these eyes are a family treasure. With a composed voice, he said it was time to make a plan. Marietta sat silent beside him, her eyes red from crying.

Like most patients initially diagnosed with cancer, he was still full of energy with all the trimmings of a good life. In my mind, I thought of the many patients I had seen die from pancreatic cancer—athletic and healthy one moment, then ravished by this cancer—often within weeks. Despite his age he hadn't slowed down by much, and he had lots of plans. Marietta had just retired from being a schoolteacher so as to have time to travel with him.

For the past two decades, I had been an oncologist, mainly taking care of patients with advanced cancer. I had spent years finding the right words for the fine line between hope and reality, guiding patients to make the choices that are right for them even when the outlook is grim. No matter how seasoned and caring, doctors are not perfect. We have limits of emotional capacity and time; and being human, we have better and worse days. Often to retain composure, we hide behind facts and technical terms. Even with patients who are not as close one's own father, it takes a toll to stay in a difficult conversation and not get overwhelmed from the suffering we see our patients go through. By nature, I am a hopeless optimist and rarely willing to give up on anyone.

But my father was then looking at me for guidance as both a doctor and a daughter. He had heard Dr. Schmied and his long-term friend and gastroenterologist agree on his prognosis of six to twelve months—at best. He had recently seen a friend die from pancreatic cancer. I knew he knew the truth, and it was my job to not cloud his vision with lies no matter how well intentioned.

For most patients, pancreatic cancer progresses very fast. It is often associated with a blockage of the common bile duct that then, in turn, chokes off the liver with bile and causes liver failure and rapid death—or even worse, it grows into the solar plexus and causes grave pain. Almost all patients rapidly lose weight and become cachectic—starved by the cancer.

We also knew that in my dad's case, surgery was not an option and the rigorous chemotherapy route would make the last days of his life miserable.

All of this he knew, and all of this applies. And yet, my research is focused on finding new treatments for patients with advanced cancer. In my heart, I knew there was hope. Particular for his type of BRCA-related pancreatic cancer, the circumstances could be different. If we had the courage, we could redirect this hopeless course.

As we sat in the garden with the sun shining on us, surrounded by birds humming and amid deeply colored summer flowers, I asked my father how much he was willing to endure and for how long.

He took some time to answer. He then looked at me. With those deep blues steadily searching mine, for the first time, I realized that our responsibilities for each other had changed. He was imploring me for guidance, as a doctor and as someone whom he implicitly trusted. He was not willing to give up yet, but he needed to know whether I truly believed that we could shrink his tumor.

"Is there hope and a way to shrink this tumor so I can go through surgery?" he asked.

"Yes," I said, "but it comes at a price; and at the risk that despite very aggressive chemotherapy, the treatment may not work and the tumor might continue to grow anyway."

"What will be my alternative?" he asked.

"You can hope for slower growth of the tumor and some meaningful time before the tumor creates problems. Pancreatic cancer typically grows steadily and rapidly, sooner or later will cause pain and may compromise your liver," I responded somberly.

He then asked me an even more difficult question: "Do you really think this will work?"

My father has been my stronghold all my life—tough and driven, rarely letting obstacles stand in his way. Ever since I was a little girl, he instilled in me determination and grit. He would never let me shy away from a challenge, always confident that I could do it. I could not really see him able to give up that easily, nor would I want him to.

"The odds are against you. But, knowing you, I think you would rather go down in flames than not try at all."

I looked at him and then at Marietta, garnered my courage and gave my opinion in my most assured oncologist voice: "If you were my patient, I would give you four weeks of chemotherapy and see whether you can tolerate it and whether the tumor is shrinking. If it doesn't work, we call it quits and you have given it a good fight. If it works, we see how far the tumor shrinks and hopefully get you to surgery."

Both of them nodded.

"One last question: Do you think I can do it at my age?" Dad asked.

With tears welling up in my eyes, I said with a grin, thinking of his previous comments that age is a matter of mind. "If anyone can do it, it will be you!" Marietta grabbed his hand and said, "We will all be at your side!"

Over the next days, I talked to two of my oncology colleagues with practices in my dad's town, and we worked up the treatment schedule. An intrepid young colleague, Dr. Stefan Greuter, was willing to help us despite his own logical hesitations at the idea of treating my seventy-eight-year-old father with folfirinox, a combination of chemotherapy that puts even the toughest patients at risk for severe infections, nerve damage, allergic reactions, heart arrhythmias, and much more. Only because Dad had a BRCA mutation, and an extremely persuasive daughter, did he agree to at least try this chemotherapy for one or two slightly reduced doses. He must have felt slightly more reassured upon seeing my father skip into his office to talk about the game plan. Dad really still skips when he is ready to tackle something.

Until very recently, I didn't admit to anybody, hardly even myself, just how nauseated I was watching one of the nastiest chemotherapies available today flow into the veins of someone I loved so dearly. At my instruction, my father received what can only be referred to as poison. While I prayed that it would work, I also swore I would continue to focus my career to come up with better treatments to treat this disease.

From the beginning, I had been merely hoping for a response—any response—so I was quite unprepared for the drastic changes in Dad's tumor. After two weeks, Dr. Greuter called me excitedly and told me that the tumor markers (a blood test that can tell us what the tumor is doing before we see it on a scan) had dropped from over 500 to 90—in other words, a huge drop. I made him email me the test result so I could see for myself.

By that time, I was back at work. I had received reports from Marietta: The chemotherapy was tough on Dad as predicted, but he tolerated it quite well overall and was mostly up and about the next day after chemotherapy—even fixing a new solar panel on his roof. Over the next six weeks, he received three more chemotherapy sessions. After the chemotherapy, the tumor was less than half its original size.

We went to see Dr. Schmied after Dad had completed eight weeks of chemotherapy. Clearly surprised to see us back in his office at all, Dr. Schmied was even more surprised to see my father's response to the chemotherapy.

"It is the BRCA mutation. These tumors are much more sensitive to chemotherapy!" I explained.

The surgeon looked at me inquisitively. "Why is that?"

"The same defect that makes people with BRCA mutations more likely to have cancer, is also the Achilles' heel of these tumors. BRCA-related cancers are very susceptible to breaks in their DNA, so when we expose such tumors to types of chemotherapy that specifically damage the tumor DNA, the tumors take a hit and cannot recover," I said, trying my best not to sound too professorial.

"Ah, indeed," he declared, still looking in amazement at first the scans and then my dad. At that time, many doctors did not know about the relationship between BRCA2 and pancreatic cancer and the excellent response some patients can have to therapy.

Dr. Schmied and his team agreed to attempt the surgery, but spent a lot of time impressing upon Dad and me how difficult it would be. Even with a good response to the chemotherapy and no visible tumor spreading to the liver or the lining of the abdomen on the scan, it was highly possible that he would cut my father open and find tumors everywhere. Small tumor seedlings are often too small to see on the most detailed of scans.

He suggested that to be prudent, he would first take Dad into surgery, open up his abdomen, and take random samples of tissue and lymph nodes in the area around the tumor. The pathologist would take samples during the surgery and check for the tumor immediately. Only if these were free of cancer would he then proceed with the goal of cutting out the entire tumor.

Just twelve weeks after his diagnosis, in late October 2013, my dad underwent the much-hoped-for Whipple procedure. And as I knew he would—as his doctor-daughter with a foolproof intuition—he came through with flying colors. Within two days he started eating, and he recovered well enough to go home after four days in the hospital. Dr. Schmied had found no tumor seedlings and managed to remove all the pancreatic cancer, quick and clean; and upon close further inspection and tests, nothing was left behind. The pathologist looked at all the surgical margins under the microscope and reported that the margins were clear; the tumor was removed while leaving a rim of healthy tissue around where it had been. However, as warned by Dr. Schmied, recovery once again would present a challenge. My father was never heavy, but had a slightly stocky build and solid muscles; he weighed 170 pounds at the start of this ordeal.

Within two weeks, he started losing weight per the usual feared side effects (he'd ultimately lose forty pounds, never to gain them back), even though he had regained his appetite after surgery and had resumed a normal diet. In fact, all he could think of was food. Yet nothing tasted good and most foods made him feel full and bloated. This was an emotional setback as much as a physical one because of his careful yet pleasurable relationship with food. Most of their food comes from Marietta's garden, and like many Swiss, he's very fond of milk and cheese—not to mention chocolates, which were a mainstay in my family's home.

The problem lay in his newly compromised pancreas. Our diet is composed of fats, proteins, carbohydrates, vitamins, and other essential nutritional elements. As part of our normal digestion, the pancreas produces enzymes that help the gut reabsorb the fat and proteins we eat; and without supplementing these enzymes, our bodies can only take up carbohydrates, while proteins and fats pass right through the bowel. The tail of the pancreas produces insulin and glucagon and keeps sugars in the blood system stable. In addition to the loss of fat and proteins, even the carbohydrates that are absorbed may not be available to the cells that require sugar, such as those of the heart and the brain. After surgery, the remaining pancreas stump may not produce enough insulin to get the sugar from the bloodstream into these vital organs. Thus, many patients will need insulin so that they don't starve, even though they are eating all the time. Dad was lucky—his remaining pancreas made enough insulin—but he was experiencing other side effects. With insufficient supplements, diarrhea can be explosive and relentless. If the pancreas supplements are too much, bloating is common. Fortunately in this case, the remainder of his pancreas made enough insulin that he didn't need any supplement. It took about four months for him to stop losing weight. It took another four months to learn how to manage his diet and find a good combination of pancreatic enzymes, vitamins, and mineral supplements so that he could at least gain some weight back. As long as he incorporates a considerable amount of carbohydrates into his diet now, he retains most of the calories. It is much more difficult to keep fat and proteins in your body after a Whipple procedure because a large section of the intestines, where proteins and fats are absorbed, have been removed. So, as do many other patients with pancreatic cancer, my dad remained insatiable and ate everything in sight. With some setbacks, he slowly regained his strength and life returned to normal. Less than a year after his surgery, we were back on long hikes in the Swiss Alps.

Two years later, in December 2015, his tumor had come back and required more treatment with another short round of chemotherapy. Again, the tumor was exquisitely sensitive and shrank briskly; but now at age eighty, he had a much tougher time of it. He recovered and got a break for seven months, requiring no therapy during that time. Then out of the blue, more tumors again came back—one blocked the drainage of the bile from the liver into his small bowel and choked off the liver. Almost from one day to the next, he turned dark yellow, his urine the color of ale. He was rushed to surgery to place a stent to drain the accumulation of bile in his liver. He had barely survived a complete liver shutdown.

Since he firmly refused more chemotherapy, Dad told us we had to come up with another plan for treatment.

His Swiss oncologist and I put our heads together and spoke with our radiation therapy colleagues. Radiation therapy is well known to cause DNA damage, so in principle, a BRCA-related tumor that cannot repair DNA strand breaks should also be very sensitive to radiation. Dad's tumor was sitting in a tight spot, though, making radiation more difficult. It took very careful planning and targeting to direct the radiation beam at only the tumor, with minimal damage to the surrounding tissue. Fortunately, the radiation worked like a charm and shrank the tumors again, and surprisingly he had virtually no side effects. Or maybe he just did not complain. We repeated the same again when more tumors creeped up eight months later.

For now, Dad is fine and enjoying what seems to be his new lease on life. Since his diagnosis, an entirely new type of therapy for BRCA-mutated tumors has been developed and approved, so if more tumors crop up, we should be ready to tackle them with a better method. The discovery of the PARP inhibitors has made in an enormous difference in the lives of many patients with ovarian cancer–related BRCA mutations, and if the tumor will grow back yet again, the next step for him will be a PARP inhibitor.

Unfortunately, the story of my dad has not been the story of most patients with pancreatic cancers. As he goes for his follow-up appointments, he is not oblivious to the surprised glances of nurses and doctors who marvel at the response of his tumor.

"People look at me as if to say, 'Why are you not dead yet?'"

"Surely, no one would say that," I retort, but from the looks he gives me, I gather he is not entirely off the mark.

Much of my dad's story is about what being at the forefront of medical research did for him; he was lucky his BRCA mutation was recognized. Hopefully, in the very near future, with increasing awareness, many more patients will benefit from similar research and new treatments. I am lucky to have had many more years with my father since his diagnosis than originally predicted, and this gift has propelled me to keep faith in research and solidified my steadfast belief that there is always hope. But I could not end his story without reflecting upon what *he* did to make this happen.

Dad was seventy-eight when diagnosed. Until then, he had exercised most every day of his life and ate a balanced diet. These facts may not have prevented his tumors from growing, or occurring in the first place, but they clearly helped him to survive the blows of treatment.

A friend once told me that to win the race you had to stay in the race. Dealing with metastatic cancer is an ongoing war. It requires support, resources, stamina, and most of all, courage and hope. There are endless setbacks and bad days. In fact, it is important to come to terms with the fact that there will be *many* bad days. Having been given extra days does not mean they will all be ecstatic and blissful. For every cancer patient, the new norm is to sometimes feel moody, tired, or even hopeless.

There were many days when things were rough. Even though he seemed to have minimal side effects, the chemotherapy caused fatigue and made his skin raw. No one can know when their last day will be, but for a cancer patient with metastatic disease, death is always on the horizon of tomorrow. And anxiety in men often turns into anger and irritability.

Marietta has been on his side for all of these days, steadfast and forever with understanding and a smile. When he gets really morose, we remind him *and us* of the good days. And more often than not, making a chocolate cake has rescued the day.

Watching him, I am so proud. I cannot help but go back to my work—to study harder and make it a bit better for my patients, all of whom are somebody's mother or father, daughter or son.

I know it will take a while before we can get everyone tested for their risk for pancreatic cancer, and then work on the best ways we can truly prevent pancreatic cancer and make preventive surgery easier. However, we do know now how to test and screen women for breast cancer and how to prevent a disease that still claims so many lives, when just like in my case, this could have been entirely preventable. Because of our circumstances I was able to influence Dad's course. In the first weeks after his surgery, we talked about how much he would love to see my sons go to college, his granddaughter settled at least in high school. I am grateful that he got his wish, and I am hoping he will be able to see all my three kids in college. It marks the rite of passage for our children and in a way for parents: Knowing their children will be well on their way to find their own path is something almost every one of my patients wishes for.

As it was the most profound wish for Lis to see her boys graduate high school.

Chapter 11

Life After Lis:
How a Family Copes with Loss

T hree weeks before Christmas is a busy time for most high school seniors today. For the select few who have already chosen a college and placed applications for early decisions, this time is one of apprehensive waiting; for most others, it is a frantic time full of completing college applications and writing moving responses to essay prompts. Watching my oldest son put the final touches on his college application, I could not help but think how much easier life seemed when I was young. I used to love the time before Christmas, the air softly scented with the smell of cookies, a fire in the chimney lit with the sweet anticipation of the holidays. But here was my boy, now physically all grown up at seventeen, at the pinnacle of three years of hard work, suddenly up for judgment—confident and excited, but also worried, too much so to enjoy the holidays at all, swept up in the frenzy of the ever-increasing competitiveness of the process, and of life, and unable to take a few days off for family and tradition.

Seeing him desperately trying to put a nonchalant expression on his face to hide his feelings, I put my hand through his hair. And I was very deliberately not seeing the poorly suppressed flash of annoyance for the parental affection in my boy. As a mom, I would do anything to take the pressure off him. So I smiled at him and offered to read another prompt for him. He reluctantly accepted, and I sat down to read with him, hoping to ease his tension a little. Looking at his young, concentrated face, I reflected on how lucky he was, how lucky I was. My brief interaction with breast cancer was well behind me, and my father was doing well with his treatment. Tears of gratitude welled up in my eyes, as I pictured how very different this period was for David, Lis's oldest son when he was at that age. David had told me this story during one of many hours we were walking the annual thirty-nine miles, raising awareness for breast cancer on his mother's team. From being completely immersed in the application process, within one afternoon the worry about college had become much less relevant for David.

Driving home from school one early December day, David had been preoccupied trying to decide what to write about for his college essay—his love for languages, and why he wanted to major in them, or how his mother had beaten breast cancer nine years ago?

As he pulled up into the driveway, he took a moment before getting out of the car. His mother had recently had a PET/CT scan of her body because of an abnormal blood test, and the whole family was waiting anxiously for the results, hoping it wouldn't be the same as last time—that this would not be cancer. As he sat in the driver's seat, he saw his grandma come outside to look for him, obviously having heard the car pull up. Her whole body shook and her tiny, wrinkled face was ashen.

David got out of the car and walked into the house with her. Nervously she told him that his parents had driven down to the city to see a new doctor for a second opinion.

He knew instinctively that the results must have been bad, since his parents did not tell him about a planned visit as they always had. Over the past days he had been surfing the web for any possible explanation besides cancer for an abnormal scan in someone who had had cancer before. And at the same time, he was pushing himself to finish all his college essays as a gift to his mother, in case this was to be her last holiday. Now it seemed all his research had been futile, and that he should have spent more time working on that last gift for her. When he finally heard his dad's car outside hours later, he ran out anxious to see his mom and find out what the future had in store. When she got out of the car and looked at him, her eyes were tear-stained.

Meeting Lis that day for the first time as her doctor is a memory etched into my mind. I had tried sneaking out of the house early to beat traffic that morning, but I should have known I'd never outsmart my seven-year-old daughter, who ran out of the house in her pajamas to hug me good-bye. My older boys sleepily waved at me from the kitchen, having already outgrown the hugs but not the good-byes.

Despite my best intentions, it turned out to be another one of those unpredictable days, when the best-laid schedule and strong determination to stay on time fell apart. Since most of my patients have Stage IV cancer, their appointments with me are inevitably fraught with uncertainty. A visit could be scheduled for thirty minutes but turns out to need twice as much time when somebody arrives with new symptoms that need more attention. I never really know when a CT scan shows progression of someone's tumors and new treatment decisions are needed.

That particular afternoon, I remember talking to the emergency room doctor about a patient who came to the ER with an unusual side effect from an investigational drug. Impatiently standing in the hall, one of the nurses reminded me that she needed me to address a dosage question for someone else who was waiting, frustrated, in the chemotherapy infusion center for her drugs to be ready. I was desperate for chocolate and coffee—about the only thing predictable about this scenario at this time of day—but in addition to these demands I still had my last patient for the day, scheduled last-minute as an "overbook." My clinic scheduler had added her just this morning, saying she needed to be seen urgently.

Before walking into the small examination room, I had glanced at this woman's medical record. I knew she was forty-six with newly diagnosed metastatic breast cancer, recurring after almost a decade. I knocked and entered the room to see Lis, her husband, and a friend, sitting huddled together—six eyes boring holes through me with expectation. Lis was wearing a white, soft sweater and a comfortable-looking pair of slacks, her shoulder-length blond hair neatly curled. Her luminous eyes intently surveyed me, and then she bestowed that incredibly sunny smile upon me for the first of many memorable times.

Lis told me she had recently seen her doctor before being released from the oncology clinic after ten years of follow-up. The doctor had ordered a set of labs, including tumor markers to determine whether there were any tumors hiding somewhere in her body. We don't routinely recommend checking for tumor markers, as far too often they can be falsely elevated—or even still normal—in patients with documented metastatic disease. Of course, after an almost ten-year reprieve, no one really had expected this bad surprise, because the late recurrences are not as often talked about. Lis did not have any back pain, nor did she have any other noticeable symptoms or physical findings. In fact, she had no symptoms at all. She felt great and looked the picture of health. Her life had returned to normal after her initial diagnosis with breast cancer and she had been thrilled to be coming up for her tenth anniversary. By now, statistically the odds of her tumor coming back had been very low, much less than 10 percent. After all, Lis had Stage II breast cancer before, her tumor was small, and it had affected only one of her lymph nodes. She had also undergone bilateral mastectomies, four months of chemotherapy and then five years of tamoxifen—the duration for treatment that was recommended at that time. By everyone's reckoning, breast cancer was behind her and she went on with her life.

There is much talk about the five-year mark. And like many patients, she was unaware that estrogen receptor–positive tumors, such as hers, can come back late, even after many years. Contrary to either HER2 or triple negative breast cancers, which rarely come back late, if these reportedly more aggressive cancers do come back, it is usually earlier—often before the five-year mark.

When her tumor markers came back higher than expected, Lis's oncologist had ordered a CT scan and found her spine showed several abnormalities, a very suspicious development for metastases. The morning I saw her, the report of the bone biopsy had come back and confirmed the recurrence of her breast cancer just as it had been, still ER positive and HER2 negative. This now meant that she had metastatic cancer, or Stage IV. Her breast cancer was incurable whether she was originally Stage I, II, or III. When it comes to Stage IV, what matters is whether it responds to therapy and where the tumor has spread to. Some areas, such as the bones, are easier to treat and have fewer symptoms than if the cancer has metastasized to the liver or the brain.

Lis had come to me for a second opinion based on a recommendation of a friend of hers who was also my patient. As she told her story, I wondered what her life had been like prior to this morning's phone call. I glanced at her husband, a well-put-together man with a gentle face pulled taut with worry. Her friend, sitting between them, seemed genuinely supportive but overwhelmed with the news. Did Lis know about her situation, what was going to happen to her? Did she have young children? Not ready to ask these questions yet, instead I asked her what she remembered from the prior therapy.

"It was not all that bad, a bit of a blur now," she said. "I was going to work through most of it." She reflected, then added with a smile, "I hated losing my hair, and it took a long time to grow back."

After a pause she said, looking at her husband, "It was hard on my family—our boys were still in elementary school."

I nodded. Listening to this very composed-seeming person speak of tackling all the stresses of the diagnosis, of going through surgery and chemotherapy, and of keeping up with a full-time job and three preteen boys, I pictured her handling it all with grace. The early days of a breast cancer diagnosis are usually very intense, and all the focus is on getting the patient through treatment and then hopefully back to a normal life. Even when a patient is fraught with anxieties, and dealing with side effects, there is always an end in sight. Early-stage breast cancer is curable and there is a very high chance to be able to put it all behind within a few months. After going through the acute treatment phase, the doctor visits become less frequent, usually focused on the required follow-up mammograms and to discuss side effects or concerns with the hormonal therapy. Most early-stage patients come in twice a year, and the visits usually include a positive update on life—how life after cancer is evolving.

Lis's post-early-stage cancer phase had come to an abrupt end. Dealing with metastatic cancer would mean needing treatment just to keep her cancer at bay, but with little hope to ever completely eradicate it. If I became her doctor, our relationship would be much closer than the one she had with her previous doctor because she would come in for many more visits. And looking into her hopeful eyes that afternoon, I was profoundly aware that in the absence of a miracle, this relationship would end in death. This was my chance to protect myself and not get emotionally involved with her. At least, that's what I was told early in medical school training—don't get involved in patients' lives.

I decided it wasn't something I needed to think about in this case, because it was more likely that she would want to be treated closer to home, rather than driving into the city to see me. She had been seen by her local doctor for a long time. For a moment, I let misery sweep over me. How unfair life was for some. For this lovely and vivacious woman, her husband, and their three boys, from now on her life would be like flying an airplane with a broken fuel gauge. Cruising along for a time but never knowing for how much longer.

I snapped out of my sorrow and back to reality. Mustering all of my optimism, I grabbed a pen and started to gather the medical information I needed to make the best treatment recommendations for her. Had the tumor caused any symptoms at all? Had she noted maybe the slightest twinge of a side effect? Any weight loss, any change in energy level, fatigue, pain when she lifted a heavy object? I was looking for anything to give me an idea of how long the tumor had been present in her spine.

But nothing in Lis's history could give me any idea how of how fast these tumors were growing; besides, it could have taken almost ten years for the tumor cells in the spine to be big enough to be visible on scan or they could have gotten very aggressive just over the last few months. It was a good sign that the tumors did not grow during the time she took the tamoxifen, suggesting that the tamoxifen, at least while she took it— had kept the cancer at bay.

It was important that none of the tumors had metastasized to other parts of her body, such as her liver or lungs. So, hopefully, while getting her back on hormonal therapy would not keep her tumors in control forever, it would do so for a few years.

I put my pen down and leaned back in my chair. "What kind of support system do you have at home?"

Her husband said: "You are looking at it."

Lis smiled at him in a way that told me he'd be her rock.

The friend nodded. "Lis has a lot of friends. We all love her and will be there for her." Briefly, I thought of my own grandmother, and how lonely she must have felt after her diagnosis. I wish I could have been there for her. And for the many women who routinely come in alone. Lis seems lucky in that regard.

"Before I lay out the options for the best treatment, would you like to ask any questions?" I sat back, making sure to avoid naturally crossing my arms so as not to appear defensive.

She paused for a long moment, then said, "Many. But I want to wait until I hear your treatment plan, so I can be more specific in my questions.

"Your tumor has spread to the bones and is now metastatic," I said. "The cells that have settled in the bones have likely been there for a long time and have been held in check by your chemotherapy—and probably even more so with the tamoxifen. When you stopped the tamoxifen, it still took more than four years for these cells to now manifest themselves. Since you don't have any symptoms, we can't really tell how quickly these tumor cells are growing or whether they are still sensitive to hormonal therapy. Only time will tell." And then added, "However, since you're still premenopausal, I think your tumor cells are still being driven by estrogen; and so shutting down your ovaries and giving you a drug that also blocks the production of

estrogen in other tissues—an aromatase inhibitor, such as letrozole—will likely be the best options." I paused and looked to see
whether she still was with me.

"Should I have stayed on tamoxifen?" she asked.

I lowered my head, wishing I could avoid an answer I never
liked giving—that knowledge has evolved and we have better
treatment now, but that knowledge is too late for the person
in front of me. "We now know that staying tamoxifen for ten
years is better. But at the time you finished your five years of
tamoxifen, we did not know that. We also can't know whether
staying on the drug longer would have made any difference."

She seemed consoled by the fact that she had had the best
treatment option then.

"More importantly, however, we have a new treatment that's
given with hormonal therapy. This new class of drugs, the
CDK4/6 inhibitors, block the cells from growing in a different
way and together with hormonal therapy that blocks estrogen
receptor signaling, the benefits of this combined therapy last
almost twice as long. This therapy is usually well tolerated,
and it should keep your tumors under control for a long while.
Because there are several areas of tumor in the spine, there's
greater risk that the treatment will shrink the tumor tissue
and the bone. So, it also would be wise to give you a bone
strengthener, to prevent fractures if a tumor causes any weakness in one of the bones. We have now several drugs to prevent
fractures that are usually given monthly as an IV infusion or an
injection in addition to the treatment for your breast cancer."

Lis asked, "Why is this better than chemotherapy?"

"It took a long time for the tumors to grow back after you stopped the tamoxifen—what we call disease-free interval. This tells me that the tamoxifen worked. Hence I am hoping that it still will work when we restart. Whether it works better than chemotherapy, we will find out after we start, but it is much better tolerated than chemotherapy, and unlike chemotherapy, hormonal therapy can be taken for much longer."

"What do you mean by 'longer'? I took it for six months last time," she responded, not understanding.

"Since we cannot cure metastatic cancer and the goal is to keep the tumors from growing, we need to find ways to treat you continuously with medicines that are tolerable and allow you to have as few side effects as possible so you can go on with your life," I added gently, knowing there are no good ways of breaching the topic of incurable cancer and lifelong therapy.

"What about immunotherapy?" she asked, adding that all her friends had urged her to ask this question. I wasn't surprised as immunotherapy has been hailed as the new cure for cancer and was everywhere online and on cancer forums. It's true there had been incredible advances in treating cancer with immuno-therapy—just not yet for breast cancer.

I tried to explain the more nuanced scenario of this treat-ment. "Immunotherapy engages your own immune cells to eradicate cancer cells. There has been great success with this type of therapy in many tumor types, with amazing responses in melanoma and lung cancer. But somehow, unlike melanoma and lung cancer, breast cancer cells don't seem to stimulate a strong immune response in patients, which makes it harder to engage immune cell to kill tumor cells. So far, immunotherapy is still experimental in breast cancer. If the hormonal therapy does not work, I will try to get you enrolled on a clinical trial testing immunotherapy and maybe by the time you need different treatment, immunotherapy has become standard therapy for breast cancer."

Abruptly I stopped myself, realizing that I went into my "professorial" mode, and smiled reassuringly at Lis and her husband. "We will always give you the best options we have at that time."

She had a few more questions and was slightly apprehensive, but warm and open. She then paused for a bit, and bestowed on me that radiant smile that would become so much part of every visit. Confidently, she told me that she would defer to my opinion and do what I thought would give her the best chance to survive this as long as possible.

"Have you told your kids yet?" I asked her as she was about to leave. As a mother of young children, this was my least favorite question to ask, unsure myself—then—of what I would say and how I would ease their fears of losing their mother.

"We told our boys that there was an abnormal scan, and that she had a bone biopsy. Our visit today has now confirmed the recurrence of her tumor." Both Lis and her husband looked at me. "How much more should we tell them?"

"It's a difficult question and there is no right or wrong answer," I replied. "This very much depends on your level of comfort, their maturity, circumstances. Looking at the both of you, I would think your children are very perceptive and will pick up very quickly that something is wrong. It may be better if you steered the conversation and shared what you can, rather than having your children hear bits and pieces in school or via their friends' mothers. I would worry that hearing the news from friends and neighbors will make it so much worse, and it will erode their trust. And in the absence of information, your children may think that your situation is so much graver than it really is right now. Most important, reassure them that you are going to be fine for now. In my opinion, children and young adults can handle much more than we think, and don't want to be shut out. But then again, every child is different and your oldest may already have read every piece of research about breast cancer, whereas your youngest is given his age likely at a different level."

Lis nodded, and her husband explained, "We have always talked about everything in this family. I don't think we would be able to keep this a secret from the boys even if we wanted to."

Over the years of taking care of their mother I had many occasions to talk to their three children, and they always knew where she stood in her treatment. Mostly their mom would just tell them, in words or her expression, but they also gleaned information from hushed conversations from other family members and friends. David always knew that she would die, that the worst news would come. On days he knew that she had yet another scan and worried about therapy not working, he would come home and sit in the driveway for a while to find the courage to go in and get ready for the news. And then when things were fine, it was out of sight and out of mind.

I asked the youngest son, Andrew, later whether it would been easier for him to know less. He looked at me with utter disbelief: "No, I always wanted to know, needed to know where things stood. I would not have wanted to miss any time that I had with mom." His parents always shared with him what was happening, all the research studies she participated in, her optimism and later her setbacks.

As Lis and her husband were leaving, I gave her a hug. Walking down the hallway, she turned around and asked whether she could transfer her care to me.

"Of course, I am happy to take you on as a patient," I said.

Once they and their friend were out of sight, my nurse, Tara, looked at me and said, "This one is going to be hard."

"Yes, but can I really help it?" I answered, sobering at the thought.

When I was a young medical student in Switzerland, we were given well-meaning advice to avoid getting too close with patients and were cautioned about getting burned out by the relentless tragedies of their lives. Over the years, the same question has been posed by friends and strangers in different variations: *Why would you want to be an oncologist? How can you handle all that tragedy?*

Professionally I knew that Lis would die, but in all the years, my optimism to find that extra time for someone to extend their life, lessen their suffering just a bit, and then once in a while to see the miracle happen, has never left me.

But during the early years of my medical training, I often struggled with my feelings, and sometimes found myself unexpectedly angry and short tempered. It took me years to understand that when I suddenly turned irritable with a patient, my gut instinct was actually warning me that things were about to get worse very quickly. All the while my mind was still trying to hold on to the thought that I could save my patient, emotionally things would begin to unravel.

In the beginning, I tried to hide it: my sorrow, my frustrations, my anger, and most of all, my tears. I tried to protect myself, consciously or not—but there was no one to give me advice on how to find the right balance. There is no "getting used to" coping with tragedy. Losing anyone is difficult; losing someone close unbelievable.

Over the years, I have learned to forgive myself for not being able to save everybody, so I no longer consider losing a patient a personal failure. I know now that what is needed more than a cure for disease is my being present and trying my best. It's only in forgiving myself this way that I can devote my energy and training to finding new therapies for patients. I need it to maintain the confidence that for every year that I can keep someone alive, there is an increased chance that advances in medical research will give them new reasons to hope, as they did for Lis.

A few weeks later, Lis came to her clinic appointment alone and asked me my second-least-favorite question that almost always comes up over the course of an illness: "How much time do I have left?"

Even after so many years of practice and all the information we have now, I really don't the answer. We still don't have good criteria and predictive factors that tell us which tumors are very sensitive to therapy. So, it is truly impossible to predict *who* will respond to a particular therapy and *for how long*. For someone like her, whose tumor expressed ER positive and has had a long period of break, the chance to respond to the proposed therapy was about 50 percent. In the average patient, the tumors would shrink or be kept at bay for about sixteen months, some longer, many shorter. When the first therapy stops working, we start another therapy—often the medication works on the second round, but usually the duration in which the treatment works becomes shorter. The main goal and purpose of research is to find new medications so as to not run out of options.

We usually check tumor growth by a CT scan every two to three months. In breast cancer, tumors rarely go away completely, and so most patients really live from scan to scan, always with the worry that the next scan will show progression with tumors' either getting bigger or spreading to more other places.

I could tell Lis all these estimates, but the only honest answer I had was "I don't know." She prodded me for an honest guess, but my reply of "years" seemed unsatisfactory to her. I held her frustrated gaze, silently imploring her to leave it at that.

I assumed Lis had already read everything about metastatic breast cancer. Not that long ago, and as is still a preferred practice in many cultures, doctors would not even tell patients that they had cancer or that they could die from the disease—no longer the case with readily available electronic medical information. Considering that so much dubiously reliable information is available to patients, it'd be hard to imagine that she hadn't oscillated between hope and profound despair when reading about her own odds.

When she asked me to guess *and* be honest, I knew it was in part her wanting to know what her fate would be, and in part her gauging my ability to be honest and level with her. Unfortunately, I do not have a poker face and I find it impossible to lie. I have struggled with myself and in endless conversations with other professionals, often from other medical disciplines, such as palliative care service, over what the right approach to the truth should be. For me, the struggle has always been not let "honesty" extinguish hope.

I still have the very vivid memory of telling the "truth" to a beautiful young women I treated early in my career. Her name was Amy; she was a mother of a five-year-old, a college professor who had read everything about breast cancer. She had insisted that I be honest with the statistics—insisted that she needed to know how much time she had. She wanted to make plans and be prepared, she had told me. And she had the right to know, didn't she? I also had assumed that since she was informed about breast cancer, she was well aware that her chances of survival were really poor.

The statistic for women with her type of breast cancer at that time had been twelve to twenty-four months. For her particular situation, however, it more likely would be barely twelve months. But that sounded so awful for this young mother, so I had said *two* years. I had felt troubled about exaggerating by so much, and felt even worse when I saw her face erupt in devastation.

At thirty-six, two years did not feel like much to her. And they weren't, neither for her nor for her five-year-old. No amount of honesty would ever make up for this.

She did die before end of the twelve months, and all through those twelve months I cared for her, she could never regain any hope that she could be fine even for a while. My honesty had completely crushed any thought of a miracle.

I learned then what the term *brutally honest* truly meant. I pledged that I never wanted to convey this kind of hope-defeating honesty again—or be on the receiving end of it.

A hospitalist, a member of the medicine team who in many hospitals take care of our patients when they are admitted, once asked me not to give my patients more false hope, but after almost twenty years of taking care of dying patients, I ardently believe that there is no such thing as *false hope*—there is only *hope*. Until a discussion about end of life is absolutely necessary, until its omission would be misleading or would prevent a patient from making good choices, I remain optimistic and hopeful.

I'm not exaggerating when I say I've seen many miracles in patients with cancer. Every time deep despair over the relentless tragedy tries to stamp out hope, I think of my patient Ella, who had just adopted a newborn when she was diagnosed with metastatic disease. And how, during her recent visit with me eighteen years later, our discussion covered not only a promising new treatment strategy for her, but also the pros and cons of early decisions and the stress of college applications. Both of our sons would go off together, each to a different college on the East Coast.

Life is hard, but more often than not completely surprising.

So, on that day, when Lis asked me "the question," I asked her what she was hoping for.

"To get my boys through high school, get them ready for college."

"Then that is what you will do," I said confidently as I stood up. "I will never lie to you, but I will evade questions I don't have a good answer to. I am your doctor, but I am also just a normal human being with no psychic powers."

She laughed and left my office.

Watching her leave, little did I know that she would become one of my major sources for coping with my own disease. Through the years, we would have many conversations about life and living with uncertainty.

For a long time, Lis responded well to therapy. Her course during the time of her first therapy was straightforward: She had her ovaries shut down and then surgically removed and was taking an aromatase inhibitor every day. For her, these medications brought very few side effects. Even going into menopause early appeared fairly easy for her. To begin with, she had no symptoms from her tumors, and under the treatment, they had stopped growing; her scans were stable. She would need to come in only every four to six weeks, and she was working full-time. Slowly she settled into the diagnosis. She always knew in her mind that she would die from the disease, that her plane would run out of fuel. Yet, through all the years, somehow she could put that thought aside, and she *lived* until the day she died. One of the most incredible feat is having the ability to gather the strengths to enjoy the good days and be mindful of the time. Lis was a natural at staying afloat in a storm, and she made a daily conscious effort to be aware of it.

Whenever I saw her in the office, what I really wanted to know was, "How do you do it? How do you not despair when you know that your wonderful life will come to an end, and that you know that you will leave those great boys behind?"

Her secret was that she never let the thought that she would die enter her mind. Andrew told me later that until the very end, he always believed in the miracle because she instilled that hope and confidence in all of them.

And it was not that she was not aware of her situation; she remained keenly in tune with medical research and was always informed when she asked questions. It was three years into her diagnosis when her questions turned darker—to dealing with her own loss. We sat on the edge of the pool at the hotel where we stayed after a medical lecture I had given to patients and advocates. We had long become close and Lis was a fervent supporter of my research. The sun was blazing hot that afternoon with a soft, cooling breeze, one of the absolutely gorgeous fall days that make California famous.

Dangling our legs in the cool water, Lis touched my feet with hers and looked at me with her luminous greenish-blue eyes. "How do you do it?"

"How do I do what?" I asked her, dreamingly glancing over the glowing hills in the Napa Valley.

"Getting close to me, knowing that I am going to die? Why don't you protect yourself better? Are you not worried that you will burn out?"

Taken abruptly out of my daydreams, I was dumbfounded by the unexpectedness of the question. Of course, I worried. There has been many a moment over the years when I think with despair that I cannot do this another day. The days when I long to become an interior decorator and my biggest worry would be to find that a perfect orange pillow to match a blue sofa.

Looking back at her, I thought about her question and then how to find the words to express what I felt. She sat next to me, relaxed, indulgently letting the sun shine on her face. I loved her face, her sunny smile, her unwavering optimism and profound strength.

I thought about the void her death would leave in me. And then about all the many things that caring for her had given me.

Despite her having to deal with her disease, she always had encouraging words for me. During the times I was trying to cope with a disease I am an expert in, she had gentle advice for me. She was the person I would call when I could not stand another day of struggling with the uncertainties of how to pick the optimal implant size. She would then go and research implant sizes, brands, and options. She came back with detailed information and sound counsel.

After I was done with surgery, we went out to dinner. Even now a giggle bubbles up my throat when I think about our coming out of the same bathroom stall at that fancy restaurant in San Francisco, after she inspected the work of my plastic surgeon.

When I learned about my BRCA mutation, I called Lis and asked her how I would be able to handle losing my ovaries and dealing with the fear of dying of cancer. After remarking on the irony that I, the thief of innumerous ovaries, would have to ask such a question, Lis tenderly and with great knowledge walked me through all the details of side effects as they are experienced by patients, not explained by a doctor. Seamlessly, we often would switch our roles.

Slowly and inextricably, over the years, like so many I had become a member of the Lis fan club. I got to watch her manage one of the most successful Avon fund-raising teams, making the most reluctant people walk to raise money for the cause. How she relentlessly focused on advances and research, talking to the Avon folks to give me more exposure in talking about clinical trials and patients with metastatic breast cancer. Her profound strength had become contagious. I remember her walking the thirty-nine miles despite raw feet and indescribable pain that her therapy that year had given her, and still it was she who managed to encourage others on the way. All my appointments with Lis were lessons on how to handle adversity. Lis taught me how truly courageous people leverage their spirit and handle even the most vicious brutal punches. She shared the high points with me and let me guide her through the bad.

With Lis, I never worried what to say as a doctor. She faced every struggle with the one clear question, "Where do we go from here?" Lis made me a better physician and I learned that loving an exceptional person, even if only for a little while, will not make me shatter; and most of all, she taught me that being close with a patient does not make me a lesser physician.

I always knew her death would be devastating, but her unwavering support to thrive for more even if it seemed difficult or hopeless carried me through the difficult days. How could anyone want to miss out on that?

Two weeks before Lis died, her husband, Mike, asked me to come for a family meeting. Lis was feeling pretty weak and had slept most of the afternoon. Mike was worried that she was getting confused and things were taking a turn for the worse. It was late in the evening, and her sons, brother, and parents had gathered at the house. I typically don't make house calls for patients, but Lis was different.

It took me about an hour along a mostly traffic-free highway to make it up to their home on a dark October night. All along the way I was imagining what I would do when I got there. There are many outcries about oncologists' using every possible treatment we can think of and never stopping therapy—thus not giving patients the chance to die with dignity. For a long time as I was treating her, no one would ever have suspected that Lis had cancer, or even metastatic cancer. She was always fit and radiant. I had many conversations with her about her wishes and her philosophy on treatment, and about the so ominously used medical term *goals of care*. Her take on cancer therapy was that as long as I had reasonable hope to find something that could work, she wanted to try anything—approved therapy, experimental therapy on clinical trials, whatever I thought was promising. She was an educated participant in every treatment decision and usually aware of the most recent advances in breast cancer. And surely friends and well-meaning acquaintances had provided a barrage of all the nonmedical opinions and cures the web freely had to offer. She had an open mind and I knew she believed instinctively that I would always try my best for her—that I would be honest with her when the time came.

As I thought back to all the conversations I had with Lis about her treatments, I now wondered whether I'd done the right thing. Had I given her enough opportunities to stop therapy over the last few months, as the treatments had become difficult? When she would report that she could barely tolerate the pain or was really fatigued, I usually would counsel her to take more pain medication and rest. Should I have offered more adamantly for her to stop then?

Andrew told me later that the day I came up was one of the worst days of his life. He was in the room when Mike was talking with me on the phone, and he overheard the conversation that I was worried his mother may not make it through the night.

Just before I got there, Andrew was sitting at Lis's bedside, when she woke up. She looked at him confused and asked him what was wrong, not understanding what was happening to her. Her failing liver made her drift in and out of consciousness. His heart broke, knowing that he knew more about her condition than she did and feeling that he had completely led her down.

By the time I got to the house, Lis was in the bedroom, awake and temporarily very clear in her mind. It's not uncommon for a patient's alertness to wax and wane at this stage. She took my hand and looked at me, the question burning in her face: "Is this it?" With tears in my eyes, I just looked back at her and nodded imperceptibly.

She closed her eyes without saying anything further. Tears silently ran down her cheeks. When she opened her eyes again, she told me that she wanted to go and meet the family in the living room. I helped her out of bed and we walked to the living room, where her parents and brother were sitting on the sofa.

Her brother rushed to get her a glass of water, a blanket, and a pillow.

All eyes were directed expectantly at me. I sat next to Lis and remained quiet, anticipating what would happen next.

Gathering all her strength, Lis told her mom and dad that this was just a bit of a downturn, but that I would get her on another treatment and she would be better soon. The family looked at me with such profound relief that I could only nod. Mike stared at me, dubious, but Lis just smiled her angelic smile. She was not ready to give up.

After her parents left, Lis told me she wanted to go back to bed. I hugged her and bade her farewell, and on the way out I whispered to Mike that I would call him from the car.

As I was getting ready to leave, David appeared and asked me whether I would talk to him, alone. We sat out on the steps for a long while looking at the brilliant stars in the night sky. Silently crying.

"What will happen?" he finally asked me. I knew he had recognized Lis's heroic effort to again put everyone at ease.

"Her liver is failing and she will very gradually get more and more sleepy and more confused. In between, she will sometimes be very clear. During these moments, you will need to tell her that is okay for her to let go, tell her how much you love her and that you will be okay," I said gently.

One of the cruelest trials for my young mothers and fathers with cancer is the thought that they are abandoning their children, failing the most primal duties in life, protecting their children. I have seen mothers take on the most enormous challenges, to be there for the kids. Lis's cancer journey had started when her youngest was three years old. Her goal when she came to me was to see her boys through high school and to college. The night I came to see Lis, Andrew finalized his college application that was due the next day. While traditionally Lis would have been the final editor, this night she lay sleeping on the other side of the wall that separated the kitchen from the master bedroom. In her place, her husband, her brother and sister-in-law, and her oldest son, David, filled in as the editing team. The application wasn't to be submitted until each person had signed off on each essay. At 3:00 am Andrew hit the Submit button.

Eight months later, I walked my fifth Avon Walk with Lis's family, no longer a team survivor but in her honor. Mike told me a story from the night she passed away. He and his three sons had gone for a hike on the mountain behind the family home. The hike had two purposes: to honor Lis's love of hiking, and to symbolically put one foot in front of the other and keep moving, as she would have wanted for them. The destination was the Wishing Tree, a lone magnificent eucalyptus tree that stood atop the mountain—and the family had plenty to wish for. As they walked lost in thought, day turned to night. Along the way, Mike and his sons stopped at a large climbing rock that offered views of the twinkling lights of San Francisco. They rested on top of the rock and reflected at what they'd all just experienced. At times they sat in silence, deep in their own thoughts. And then softly speaking into the darkness, Mike brought up an exchange that he and Andrew had had a few weeks earlier. Walking out from the ICU, Andrew had stopped Mike and asked, "Dad, what are we going to do?"

the implication being without Lis. Caught off guard by the question, Mike responded, "I don't know; we're going to have to figure it out."

Sitting on the rock after saying good-bye to her, Mike asked, "Andrew, do you remember the question that you asked me a few weeks ago?"

Andrew replied, "Yes."

Mike continued, "I think it's the wrong question. I think the right question is, 'What are we going to do with everything that Mom taught us?'"

Walking alongside Mike on the Avon walk, I closed my eyes and thought about Lis and all she taught me.

Lis never knew what caused her cancer; she did not have a BRCA or any other cancer mutation. She had done everything possible to survive her disease, and in the end she did not. However, the life and death of Lis, and so many men and women like her, who with their courage and poise make us better doctors, impact research, and teach us to love even if time is short. They are the people who make me want to continue and not give up hope that each year, life with cancer becomes a little more hopeful, a little less painful. I always miss her, but not for anything would I want to have missed having her in my life.

Chapter 12

The Gift of BRCA:
Getting Tested for Cancer Mutations

If there is a silver lining to having a BRCA mutation, it could be considered an *unappreciated gift*. If Lis had a daughter, I could not predict what her risk for breast cancer is. This is much different for Meghan.

Meghan, age thirty-six, had come to clinic to offer moral support to her thirty-eight-year-old sister, Kate, whom I met a few weeks earlier. Kate had presented with a large cancerous mass in one breast and sought me out to discuss treatment options. Like many patients, Kate or her sister didn't really know much when it came to family history. Their mother was fifty-seven and healthy, and they were unaware of anyone else in the family who had had cancer. They were estranged from their father, but their mother had found out that he had died in his late forties of gastric cancer: a cancer we do not typically associate with either BRCA1 or BRCA2. From what they could tell, the grandparents from the father's side were both alive and cancer-free. After Kate's diagnosis, they had probed a bit deeper in the family history of their father, but there was no report of anyone with either breast or ovarian cancer.

Since Kate was only thirty-eight at the time of her breast cancer diagnosis, she was considered a high-risk case who warranted genetic testing for BRCA and about thirty other genetic mutations; by then it had evolved into a simple saliva test we did right in my office. I was silently hoping that a BRCA mutation or another hereditary mutation might explain why she had breast cancer at this young age. At least it would help with the question that I knew Meghan would ask, and likely was part of why she came along with Kate. *What about me? What is my risk?*

When a person has a hereditary mutation in the germ cell that is passed on from either both or one parent, it's present in every cell. And since saliva contains sufficient cells shed from all the mouth tissues' cells, a small amount (about a teaspoon) is all that's needed to run the tests. There are now several commercial genetic testing companies that provide results in about two to four weeks. Unlike at the times of my testing, most insurance companies now pay for the test for women with breast cancer; and even if not fully covered, the tests are much more affordable.

Since she lived two hours away, Kate had started the chemotherapy for her breast cancer with an oncologist closer to her home, two hours away from our office. And she had already completed most of her chemotherapy cycles. So, on this day, the sisters were in the clinic to discuss her response to the chemotherapy and the results of the BRCA test.

Upon examination, the large tumor in Kate's breast was barely palpable, and the lymph nodes under her armpit had disappeared. The chemotherapy had drastically shrunk her tumors. Although she had lost her hair and was struggling with nausea, she otherwise seemed in good spirits. This great response to therapy made me suspect even more that she did indeed have a BRCA mutation.

"Is it gone?" Kate asked when I gave her the good news of the tumors' shrinkage.

My face must have completely lit up with happiness and I nodded enthusiastically. Even after so many years of seeing women with breast cancer responding to chemotherapy, the sense of profound relief when the therapy works never leaves me. And for all that medicine has done to save and extend lives, I'm always hoping that this woman will be among the last to receive it—that at some point, we will not need this type of treatment anymore and can spare women all the side effects that come with chemotherapy. One of the great satisfactions of working as a researcher and physician is knowing that there is so much progress constantly occurring all around you; that there are so many scientists around the world working endlessly to find better treatments. This was a clear sign that she had a high chance of beating this cancer.

But still, Kate anxiously searched my face for hidden worries or concerns. I smiled back at her reassuringly and she finally relaxed a little once I finished my exam. It was very obvious that Meghan, too, was extremely relieved by the good result, but she was also very apprehensive about the pending results from the BRCA testing.

Before I even managed to sit back down into my chair, Meghan blurted out, "Are the tests back? Is it bad?"

I knew that the genetic counselor had received Kate's results that morning: positive for BRCA1; we had discussed her case at the genetic tumor board. I picked up the phone and asked Julie, the genetic counselor who saw Kate at the last visit, to join me for the visit and the discussion about the results. In most centers, it's still very common that a genetic counselor who conducts testing also spends some time with the patient before getting tested, discussing what testing means and some of the consequences that a positive test could bring. However, not all centers have a sufficient number of genetic counselors on staff to see every patient. During the last visit, Kate had spent some time with Julie, discussing what a positive result would mean.

Before Julie stepped in the room, Kate cleared her voice and admitted that she only very vaguely remembered anything Julie had said in their discussion. "I know you talked to me about it, too," she said. "But I was so focused on starting chemotherapy, I don't think I heard anything of what you said."

I smiled knowingly, forever remembering my own first visit with the plastic surgeon and how little I could absorb. I clearly remember that during my first visit, I had had asked Dr. Sbitany to describe the surgery in detail. But when his first sentences described the incision with the scalpel, all I could picture was an enormous knife slicing through my chest. After that, my brain caught fire and all of the expertly explained details of the surgery were suffocated in smoke. Even after he explained it more than once, I couldn't get past that image of the knife.

There are plenty of research reports describing how difficult it is for patients to stay focused after hearing something distressing—adrenaline and cortisol surges that come with stress interfere with focus and memory. And I could neither focus nor remember. Of course, I was never really able admit to anyone how scared I actually was. Debbie, our seasoned surgical nurse, literally made me write out a list of questions to ask and then she wrote down the answers. In follow-up visits, I came prepared with a notebook and resorted to an old trick: Over the years, I had acquired some methods to control my own anxieties and worries when patients were sad, frustrated, or even angry. To not appear shifty and disinterested, I trained myself to keep my face steady, relax my eyelids, and blink slowly. Of course, when it came to me, none of these things really worked, and surely everyone could read the distress in my face. But what really helped were the notes; and in hindsight, I probably should have asked to record the conversation. I knew better than I had before not to get frustrated when patients asked the same question over and over.

"This happens to the best of us," I reassured Kate with a rueful smile, realizing I had mentally digressed. I explained the implication of the BRCA mutation again. For now, the mutation did not require any immediate action. She needed to complete the chemotherapy first. However, I shared with Meghan and Kate that we think that patients with a BRCA mutation may have a better response to the chemotherapy—or typically, at least, a very good response. I admitted that I had already suspected that Kate had a mutation because of her excellent response to the chemotherapy. Once she had completed the chemotherapy, she and her doctors would decide on the best type of surgery for her—especially whether a prophylactic mastectomy on the non-cancer other side was advisable.

"I do think however, that your tumor was caused by the BRCA mutation, hence that suggests that other family members with the mutation may also be at risk. And you know, there is a fifty percent chance your siblings have inherited the mutation."

I looked directly at Meghan. "So, what about you? You should probably get tested at some point."

Two sets of identical, bright blue eyes stared up at me in silence. After a few moments, Meghan said that she wanted to think about it. Her sister encouraged her: "Please do it," she begged; "I don't want you to end up like me!"

They were already here in the office, and the test itself would not take that long, I argued. But Meghan was still hesitant. She looked at both of us apologetically and said, "I know I should do it, but I am just not ready. Maybe after the baby. I just would not want to worry all through the pregnancy." She sat back, resolute and visibly more relaxed. She explained that she already had two sons, ages four and six. She and her husband had been talking about trying for a third, hopefully a daughter. She had read about the mutation when the news of Angelina Jolie's mutation initially broke. She recalled that "women should wait to have the prophylactic surgeries until they are finished with child bearing. And I really would like to have a baby girl! Kate told me you had a girl after two boys," she said to me, her eyes shining with a plea for confirmation.

"Oh," I said been completely caught off guard by this turn of the conversation, "That actually changes things quite a bit; and we should have a discussion about testing you now."

For a woman looking to have children, BRCA presents a whole different set of complications. It made it more urgent for

her to be tested, because if Meghan carried the BRCA1 mutation, the baby would have a 50 percent chance for the mutation
to pass on to her.

From the bewildered look in Meghan's face, I realized that
she was not following my thoughts. Clearly, she was not yet
ready to deal with this decision. However, what we were about
to discuss would drastically impact her decisions to have that
baby girl.

I tried to get control over the pang of intense guilt that
had grabbed my heart and explained my intense reaction to
her wanting to have a baby. Like many of my patients with the
BRCA mutations who did not know about it before having children, I would have given anything to not have passed this mutation on to my children. But I'd never escape the truth that each
of my two sons and my daughter have a 50 percent chance that
they carry my fate. I still don't know which, if any, of my children may have the mutation. I desperately hope none of them
does, but it could be all three. The odds are as cut-and-dried and
equalizing as flipping a coin.

Why have I not tested my kids, especially with so many
resources at my ready disposal? From a medical standpoint,
we strongly recommend against the testing of children. Normally, there are no consequences of having a BRCA mutation
(or many others) when someone is a child. Of course, there
are exceptions, and for some mutations, such as retinoblas-
toma (RB) gene and TP53, we would test early. However, the
BRCA mutation does not cause cancer in young patients. Until
a woman with a BRCA mutation is about twenty-five, there
is really no reason for cancer screening; and for young men,

matters are even less pressing—screening for prostate cancer would not be recommended until the late thirties. So, presently, I have no medical reason to test my children and find out whether they carry the BRCA mutation.

Still, my impulse was more heart- than mind-driven when I first learned about my mutation. I was consumed by getting the reassurance that none of my children carried the mutation. The thought of my little girl going through all the surgeries I had, or dying young from breast cancer or ovarian, was unbearable. I would lay awake night after night, feeling guilty that I could have passed on the mutation to her.

What made it more difficult was how easily I could have found out. A while back, even before my own diagnosis, I had ordered the 23andMe test for myself and the family, as I wanted to know our ancestry. I had sent off my own test, but had kept the tube with the DNA sample for my daughter. For months I stared at her tube still on my desk, knowing that I all I needed to do was send it out for testing or do it in my own research lab. But how I got her test done was not the problem—what to do with the result was. If I tested her and she did not have the mutation, I could finally sleep. But what if she tested positive? I would rob her of her chance to grow up without the worry of knowing. Maybe if I knew, I could just not tell her and keep it a secret? I'd have gladly carried the burden for her, but I couldn't shake my deeply held belief that patients should be able to make their own decisions about their health, no matter what the risk or prevailing medical advice. For weeks I was in turmoil over what to do—and with each restless night, my mind grew foggier and foggier about the right move.

One voice in my head would say, "Test her, you don't have to tell anyone the results!" The other voice said, "But you can barely keep trivial secrets, and usually even give her her birthday present the night before!"

In the end I decided to wait, not only for her own sake, but for my own. I would not be able to keep this truth hidden for another twenty years until she'd be at the age to start getting tested and be screened for cancer because of my history. Then, she could make the decision herself.

Exactly six months after my own results came back, I destroyed my daughter's DNA sample. Instead, I focused more intently on my research to find alternatives to a mastectomy in young women with BRCA mutations, and in the end, knowing that my daughter may be the beneficiary of such an intervention has fueled this work over the last five years. And spontaneously, one day in the car when driving home just before she turned twelve, she told me she would want to know before going off to college, so she could be mindful of her diet. As I turned to face her, she added, "Mom, since you were in your forties when you had your breast cancer, I should be safe until my thirties, and I can start screening at twenty-five."

I must have looked completely stunned, at a loss to what to say next. "Mom, I live with two oncologists, and I pay attention! I also watched one of your YouTube videos on BRCA and screening." She flashed me an impish smile with those green eyes. So much for keeping secrets from a precocious soon-to-be teenager.

"But do you think I already have cancer?" Meghan's worried voice broke into my thoughts. "Is this why you think I should be tested now?"

No, I was glad to tell her, since the test for a BRCA mutation or any other genetic cancer mutation does not detect early cancer. In Kate's case, the mutation explained why she had cancer at such a young age, as the mutation caused an increased risk for cancer. Throughout her life, harmful breaks had occurred throughout her DNA. Such breaks occur randomly and happen to everybody, and normally the body is equipped with an army of proteins to repair such breaks. However, if not repaired properly, they can cause genomic instability and can lead to cancer. But a BRCA mutation carrier does not necessarily get cancer. Much research is ongoing to further study how exactly this happens, and what the other like likely factors are, from within the person and from the environment; all these play an important role in why some women develop cancer more often, and at a younger age. This is an intense focus of current research; and the answer is truly needed so we can better predict whether and when someone with a BRCA mutation may get cancer.

Thus, if Meghan carried the mutation, her DNA would have had sufficient breaks to put her at high risk for breast and ovarian cancer. She may possibly also be at risk for other cancers, as the mutation in her father had likely contributed to his gastric cancer; even though gastric cancers associated with BRCA mutations are rare, they do occur. She would be considered a "true positive," at *risk* for cancer, but not for a diagnosis itself. On the other hand, if she did *not* carry the mutation, Meghan's result would be a "true negative" for risk. Her risk for breast cancer would be about the same as the average women in the American population, or probably even less. She would not need to undergo the early screening studies, such as regular MRIs and mammograms, and preventive surgeries that were available for Kate had we just known earlier that she had the mutation. Knowing that Meghan had the mutation might spare her from having a Stage III breast cancer like her sister.

The legendary Leonard Cohen referred to hope in one of his songs as "there is a crack in everything." The concept of being a "true negative" is that hope—the crack where the light sneaks in. Since we assume that Kate's BRCA mutation is responsible for her cancer, those family members who don't have the mutation, would also not be at risk for such cancers. My daughter, too, could be a true negative, which I would know if I had her tested. It's a huge gift to be able to reduce the worry in so many, yet such reassurance remains completely unavailable to the family members of the more than 80 percent of young women who are diagnosed with breast cancer of unknown cause. For example, Lis had five of seven first-degree relatives with breast cancer; but in her family, there was no clear mutation. Therefore, we had no way of knowing who else in her family was at risk—or why. Thus, in families without a cancer mutation, *every* woman is at variable risk; because we have no predictive marker, we will have to screen all the related females for breast cancer and possibly other cancers. In these families, we still don't really know what the right screening is, and we typically do not recommend risk-reducing surgeries, such as mastectomies or oophorectomies.

There is no best time for testing, and many people bristle at the idea of being tested for the BRCA mutation. Many fear knowing about the mutation. The actual realization of "owning" a cancer gene is likely to drastically amplify the fear of cancer, and this is especially intense in the early days after testing. And it takes some time to recognize that a 70 percent risk of having breast cancer is spread over a lifetime—it does not disappear just by knowing.

I had no real reason in Megan's case to so strongly encourage testing, and I would normally let her walk out and take her time to come to terms with the decision. But when she told us that she wanted a baby daughter, everything changed. Here Meghan had an opportunity that I and many did not have: She could stop the mutation from being passed onto her unborn children.

Interfering with nature is a difficult decision, and as my daughter once asked me, "Would you not have wanted me if you knew that I carried the gene?" Of course, I would have always wanted her, just as she is. But if possible, I also would have wanted to spare her the fears and heartache that come with carrying a cancer gene, and the knowledge of all the sacrifices she would need to make for it, and maybe someday in the near future we can do just that.

Not knowing the sisters' religious or cultural believes, I took a chance and explained this crack of hope scenario—why it was so vital to know if she was a "true negative" before trying to conceive. From their reactions, both Kate and Meghan were completely surprised by the turn of the conversation.

Kate asked, "What do you mean?" but I could tell that she was slowly realizing what I was trying to say. Since she had the mutation, she also may have passed this on to her two daughters. Her expressive blue eyes turned cloudy.

"I wish I hadn't brought this up," I said quietly, not wanting to cause Kate even more distress.

Meghan looked at me and then at Kate, confused. "Wait, no, I still don't understand."

I became deeply aware of the ethical dilemma about to play out. Torn between dropping the topic and letting biology take its course versus fully using modern technology to eliminate the mutation, I realized how much more difficult it can be in practice to guide patients through the options of interfering with genetics, than it is to discuss such ethical decisions with colleagues or at scientific meetings.

Gently I began to explain, carefully searching for the most precise words. "Meghan, I'm concerned because if you carry the mutation, you would have a fifty percent chance of passing this on to your unborn daughter. Meanwhile, there are now methods to prevent this."

"Do you mean testing my baby when I am pregnant?" Meghan asked, her posture becoming defensive.

"No, of course not; I would never suggest testing a baby during pregnancy for a mutation like a BRCA mutation," I assured her.

Her shoulders relaxed slightly and raised her eyebrows. "Then, what?" she asked, still uncertain of what I was talking about.

"We could harvest your eggs and then test embryos for the mutation before they are put back into your uterus. The concept is called preimplantation genetic diagnosis, PGD or PIGD for short. It would mean taking a few cells of an embryo that was harvested after a cycle of IVF [in vitro fertilization] and then test these cells for the mutations. If, let's say, we harvest eight embryos, four of them would likely carry the mutation, but the other four embryos would not have the faulty gene.

"Once you are ready to get pregnant, we would implant one of those four embryos that tested negative for the BRCA mutation into your uterus. This technique has been used for a few years for other mutations and has been very successful in preventing inherited diseases. These procedures are now done routinely for many patients undergoing IVF cycles. When performed early in the development of the embryo, it's usually very safe and successful."

Meghan was silent and then asked me more details about the procedures. The worst piece of the puzzle was cost, since IVF is covered in some but not all states, and pricing depends on many other circumstances. Often even with very good insurance, patients pay thousands of dollars out of pocket for the medications given during an IVF cycle and for the storing of the eggs or embryos. Given the long-term prevention of costs associated with BRCA-related cancer screening and treatment, insurance companies may be more amenable to supporting such procedures in the future, after more have reaped its benefits; many of the clinics also now have support for women without financial means.

By now, Kate and Meghan had been wiped out by this visit. I didn't blame them, so took their drawn faces as a cue to give them space. I stood up and said, "I think this is a lot for today. I am happy to see you again for further discussion."

The sisters looked at each other, and Meghan gripped Kate's hand.

"I am sorry that I am taking time away from your visit," Meghan said. Kate just gave her a smile—an expression of the love and affection that connects those to a common fate.

My hand was on the doorknob when Meghan said resolutely, "I would like to have my BRCA testing today, Dr. Munster." I turned to confirm she meant it; her eyes said it all. "Knowing will have such an impact on so many of our decisions. I just need to know!"

Within four weeks, Meghan had her results back. She tested positive for the BRCA1 mutation; and after further discussion, decided to have a bilateral mastectomy. Both she and her husband also had decided that they did not want to pursue any further pregnancies, so she also scheduled an oophorectomy within the same year, Meghan wanted to be there for her sister and her nieces during this very difficult time, and yet Kate really worried about Meghan's having breast cancer before she could get around to doing her prophylactic surgeries.

During Meghan's treatment, I had many conversations with her about her testing and shared some of my experiences. One thing she said has always stuck with me: "It's not the answer I wanted, but it was the answer I needed to make the right decisions."

As I left the clinic that night, I wondered what it would be like to be that young and have to make all these decisions. In many ways, I had been lucky because I was diagnosed when I was older. I had gone through most of my younger years oblivious to the scare of cancer—no one in my family had cancer at a young age.

Even after the discovery of my cancer and learning about my BRCA mutation, all my surgeries were done within the same year. I was not in my twenties and had to wait for year to proceed with the prophylactic surgeries. I did not (as young patients in similar circumstances have revealed), wake up in the middle of so many nights worrying about finding cancer before I'd made plans for prophylactic surgeries. Even Meghan later revealed that her own decision was prompted because she had to know for her unborn baby. It was very clear that once she knew, she felt free to act on knowledge of her mutation and move on.

For many families, the question of when to get tested remains a difficult one. After all the years that I worried what my children would do, my son decided just a couple of days after he turned eighteen.

Out of the blue it seemed, he told me that he wanted to get tested. I was surprised by his decision and double checked whether he really wanted to know.

He tossed the question back to me: "If this were you, would you not want to know?"

I looked at him, all grown up, and thought, *Yes, I would want to know for sure.*

But then, I also knew what it meant to carry this mutation, so before answering his question, I asked him what he knew about it.

He admitted that he actually knew very little, but that he had an increased risk for prostate cancer and pancreatic cancer, since his grandfather had pancreatic cancer.

"I know that had he not known about his BRCA status, Neni probably would have gotten the wrong treatment for his pancreatic cancer and be in serious trouble," he explained. "And I don't want to be in that situation—ever."

We then discussed that knowing or not at his age would not have any immediate consequences; Neni was much older and already at an elevated risk for cancer because of that. My son had years before even screenings would be recommended. However, he felt that he would change his approach to alcohol and diet, and clearly he would not smoke—as these are all risk factors for pancreatic cancer. Diet and alcohol were also risk factors for prostate cancer and male breast cancer, yet none of these cancers would be a concern for him for at least another thirty or forty years.

With a motherly wink, I pointed to the fact that he also could pass the mutation on if he got someone pregnant. Raising his eyebrows, he retorted that a pregnancy at this time of his life would have a whole set of other problems.

"True, indeed!" I replied, quickly dropping the topic. "But as much as I support you if you want to get tested, you can also wait a bit longer!"

My eighteen-year-old son did not want to wait. He wanted to know. My fifty-two-year-old brother, however, does not want to know. However, in his case, screening for all the BRCA2-related cancers, such as breast, prostate, and pancreatic cancer, would be indicated now, given his age. Starting at age forty, we would screen him for prostate cancer by a clinical exam and the PSA blood test. And, for my brother, having a father with pancreatic cancer means we would obtain MRIs or endoscopic ultrasounds for early changes in the pancreas and do a breast exam. Sometimes men (or women) really cannot tolerate the thought of knowing that they have a mutation, even if they have a 50 percent chance of having one. In such as case, even if my brother does not want to know whether he has this mutation, the medical approach to him would be to proceed with the screening procedures as if he had the mutation. In a man, the screening is typically straightforward: The PSA test is a simple blood test, and men can do a breast exam alone and consider a mammogram in addition. The screening for prostate cancer and male breast cancer are both known to save lives in patients with high risk for cancer. The controversy of PSA testing in the general population does not apply to a man with a BRCA mutation and there is strong support the early screening for prostate cancer in men with BRCA mutations.

The question of what my brother should do for his pancreas screening is more complicated. Pancreatic cancer screening is much more complicated and controversial, which leads to a more complicated question: Could the cancer in our father have been prevented had he done extensive screening?

Early screening for pancreatic cancer in BRCA carriers is still in its infancy. It is not yet clear how effective screening is because both MRI and endoscopic ultrasounds can pick up abnormalities, such as localized cancer or intraductal papillary mucinous neoplasms (IPMNs). IPNMs are very early changes in the pancreas, and are believed to be an equivalent of the DCIS in breast cancer and STIC in ovarian cancer. Such lesions are much more common in BRCA2 carriers compared to the general population. And like the discussion for breast and ovarian cancer, there is much debate over when to act upon an early form of prostate cancer—what to do when you see these IPMNs. Would surgery be wiser, or should they just be watched over years? How long could a person wait? Many research laboratories are currently developing blood tests that could tell us whether someone has early pancreatic cancer, but for now by the time such blood tests are positive, the tumor may have already attained a certain size.

Prophylactic surgery is really only an option in very special circumstances, and will only be considered in those with the highest risk for pancreatic cancer with many affected family members. Even then, most surgeons would be extremely reluctant. Removing the pancreas is technically very complicated and challenging for many reasons, not the least of which is that it is very poorly located in the body right in the middle of the abdomen, wrapped with layers of blood vessels, bowels, and nerves. It's also an organ of vital purpose: The pancreas converts food into fuel for our cells two ways, by producing enzymes to digest fats and proteins and producing insulin and other enzymes to regulate the blood sugar. Most patients who have had their pancreas removed struggle with maintaining their weight, and they often become diabetic. While pancreatic enzymes and insulin can be given to a patient to try to compensate for the missing pancreas, it is usually very challenging to mimic the role of this very finely tuned organ. Definitely not something to give up lightly, unless there is really strong evidence that early cancer is present. Many of these questions are hotly debated by experts and are still awaiting much more clarity from ongoing research studies.

Complicating the issues is that the risk of pancreatic cancer is not very high even for those with BRCA, and this can be reassuring for most people. However, the occurrence of pancreatic cancer over life is about two to three times higher for BRCA carriers than it is for men and women who do not carry the mutation. Another way of looking at it is that if we screened one thousand carriers over the age of fifty for ten years, we would find four instances of pancreatic cancer. But in families with a history of pancreatic cancer, there could be ten or more cases. To put this in perspective, the risk for prostate cancer for a BRCA2 carrier is about eight times higher compared to the risk for the average man.

For these reasons and more, of course, I wish my brother would get tested and then screened, but he is not unique in his approach; many brothers don't want to be tested. While there is no perfect age for men to get tested, ideally it should be before having children. If having children is not a consideration, a man can wait until age forty, possibly fifty. The number of BRCA-related tumors seen under age forty are very rare, less than ten per 100,000 men.

Hopefully, with more awareness, the social acceptance for men to be tested and undergo screening will change. Even if a man from a BRCA family does not wish to know of his mutation, having a PSA test starting at forty would probably be a good compromise. He also should know to report any masses or lumps in the breast tissue, and consider pancreatic cancer screening if there are multiple family members with pancreatic cancer. Much research is currently devoted to determine what other factors influence the cancer risk in a mutation carrier.

So really, I should have been happy that my son was being proactive. No matter what the test results, his adopting a lifestyle of a good balanced diet, lots of exercise, and not smoking will go a long way toward leading a healthy, cancer-free life.

The decision to get tested is different for female family members. The question of testing becomes complex when a mother with breast cancer does not want to get tested, as it will leave her daughter with much uncertainty. Testing the daughter would guide the prevention and therapy if the daughter tests positive, but it would not provide reassurance for the daughter if she tests negative. She would only be a "true negative" if she knew the mother carried the gene. And many times, the mother may have died young of breast cancer and testing is no longer possible. In this case we often try to test as many siblings as we can to determine whether the gene runs in the family.

The presence or absence of the mutation at a young age has far more implications. The female cancer rates are just so much higher than are the male cancer rates with BRCA—and they start at a much younger age. Breast and ovarian cancer in BRCA mutation carriers do occur in very young women even, college girls. My youngest patient with a BRCA2 mutation was just twenty-one at the time of the diagnosis of her first breast cancer. For most college girls, breast cancer is probably not on their minds. So, unfortunately, young women with breast cancer in their twenties are often misdiagnosed because no one would expect them to have the disease. The diagnosis and the cancer workup gets delayed, which can make the treatment itself much harder than it could be, or lead to advanced cancer when it could have been stopped early.

Women who know that they carry this mutation are typically very vigilant about their health. They don't ignore lumps or changes; and so, we often find tumors when they are still small. Many tumors present themselves between screening studies, such as in the thirty-three-year-old woman whom I saw last week in clinic. Because she knew she had a BRCA1 mutation, she went straight to the doctor's office the same day she felt a lump while taking a shower. She saw a surgeon and had a biopsy and an MRI all within a few days. It was a cancerous tumor, but luckily for her, it was still Stage I. Four months earlier, she was completely fine; her screening MRI had been normal. And when all of a sudden the lump came up, it was still a shock but it did not come as a surprise and she knew what to do about it. All too often, we see young women in our practice who had felt a lump and not know how to act. And it often takes a woman some time to find a doctor and get a diagnosis. Fortunately, not every lump is a tumor.

There are other preventative measures patients can take once they know their mutation status. For carriers, it's been proven that birth control pills protect against ovarian cancer; although they may increase the risk for breast cancer slightly, the benefits in the protection of the ovaries trump the risk for breast cancer. We would start screening a young woman for breast cancer with an MRI at age twenty-five at least once a year and then get mammograms with it. The risk for ovarian cancer starts rising after age forty for BRCA1 carriers, and later in BRCA2.

The timing for removing the ovaries involves many factors: Are there other family members with ovarian cancer? How old was the youngest family member at time of diagnosis? Has the person completed child-bearing? Should embryos and eggs be harvested? What is the risk for other illness such as heart disease, or the risks of compromising bone health? Since there may be a negative effect on the overall health of a young woman who is going into menopause in her early thirties, we like to wait until her late thirties. Many ovarian cancers start in the endings of the fallopian tubes, so more and more surgeons have started to remove the tubes in a BRCA carrier, to delay surgical menopause a bit longer.

Nonetheless, it is difficult for my twenty-eight-year-old patient with Stage I breast cancer, whose mother died of ovarian cancer in her early fifties, not to worry about ovarian cancer. Her mother also had breast cancer when she was young, just thirty-three. For her, removing her fallopian tubes is an intermediate option, since after breast cancer, oral contraceptives are no longer an acceptable. The goal of treatment for a breast cancer is to withdraw estrogen and progesterone, just the opposite what oral contraceptives do. Living with a mutation is in no way easy, but it allows a young woman control—and hopefully, prompt medical care.

While testing itself was a major barrier for many years, my children's generation will grow up with much more information about their genetic makeup than we had. Genetic testing is rapidly become available everywhere and affordable. The FDA recently approved 23andMe as the first consumer-directed genetic testing panel that allows anyone with a credit card to order their genetics. As part of the gene panel, select BRCA1 and BRCA2 mutations are reported back to anyone who buys this test. However, so far the BRCA testing only includes the mutations found in Ashkenazi Jewish families. And so 23andMe had not picked up my BRCA mutation. Until recently, online tests included genetic counseling as part of the testing kit and usually required the name of a doctor (as a consult) to be listed.

The technical challenges and costs for genetic testing have long been solved, but there are still major challenges regarding the impact of this knowledge. We may have access to a piece of our fates, but we still don't know for sure what a mutation really means for an individual and how it impacts risk for cancer or even other diseases.

These and other unknown questions are bubbling to the surface very quickly as we do more work in this field. If a mutation is associated with cancer, meaning it's pathogenic, it predisposes cells to turn into cancers—we just don't know how, when, or what kind. Most mutations are further impacted by environmental influences. We know about the negative role of a diet rich in red meat for colon cancer and that there is a worse outcome in women with breast cancer who are sedentary. There are the negative effects of prolonged combined hormone therapy and the detrimental effects of alcohol. We still know very little about the immune system and how the control of infections in the era of global vaccination influences the development of cancer. And just as there are genes that cause cancer, there are colliding genes that may protect against cancer.

All of these factors will have to be considered when genetic testing becomes more widely available. In the absence of a sound medical reason and a genetic counselor for guidance, people who in the spur of the moment order such a test online or get a testing kit from their friends may be exposing themselves to more than they thought.

I know how my son felt—that desperate need to know what one's body has in store for us. Yet all knowledge should be sought with guidance and expertise. No one should be out there, lost, when the result of mutation testing is ready in the inbox.

The story of my family has shown how much knowing about this mutation has done for us. My father would not have had so many extra years, and I got spared from advanced breast and ovarian cancer and hopefully will be prepared for other cancers to come. But most of all, it should give hope to all affected family members that there is so much care, knowledge, and research out there.

Research is underway from every angle. There are better treatments for those with cancer, sophisticated tests for early detection for those with the mutation, and gene selection and gene editing to prevent the mutation to be passed on to the next generation. Testing is now affordable and available for almost everybody, and several new therapies allow the specific treatment for BRCA-related cancer for those with cancer. For the next few years, finding better tests of early detection of cancer and tolerable therapy that prevents cancer from developing is well within reach, and hopefully the need for the removal of body parts will become less and less. Gene editing of the germ line and in tumors may take a few more years, both technically and emotionally.

Hopefully, for my grandchildren, my story will be part of an interesting family saga, with a medical problem from the past but not one for their present.

Afterword

My friends insist that I would never need additional preventive measures to avoid dying from cancer. Not because I'd done everything in the textbooks possible at this time, but because my lifestyle puts me in more danger than cancer ever would. In March 2018, at the six-year mark of my diagnosis, I spent five days heli-skiing in Canada. Prepared for every scenario, I carried an avalanche beacon, a radio, and a prudent head on my shoulders. I did not realize that nature may not always feel the same as I do. Skiing through dense trees with a group of skiing buddies is a particular thrill. But on this fateful run, while enjoying a particularly exhilarating moment of flying through a densely populated forest in deep power, I had to abruptly slow down to give way to a colleague who was cutting into my way. Losing speed in deep powder snow in trees, however, proved treacherous. Before I could regain my speed to clear the tight space between two trees, my skis got trapped in the heap of the snowpack that had formed outside the branches. I lost my balance and the ground gave way under me. Slowly and helplessly I fell headfirst into the twenty-foot-deep sheltered space around the low-hanging branches of tree, ominously called a tree well.

Fortunately for me, my skis got hung up in branches, preventing me from falling all the way to the bottom, so I only fell five or six feet into the tree well. My legs stuck, my left arm buried, I was effectively immobilized, but with extraordinary fortune, my right arm was free.

Having read many safety manuals and videos and talked through a hypothetical incident and mock rescues of a mountain guide, I was prepared. *Don't panic, don't wiggle, don't fall deeper! Protect your airway! Signal for help! Stay hopeful!*

But hanging upside down, inhaling a mouthful of fluffy snow, of course I panicked. I thrashed around helplessly and thought of digging myself out. Luckily, after being trapped and struggling for air for a few moments, my senses returned. No matter how scared I felt, I knew, I could do this.

Throughout my cancer I learned that there is always help out there. So, I slowed down my breathing and brought my brain into focus. Carefully I patted down snow around me to find an air pocket to breath. Once I found the calm I usually have for someone else in crisis, I looked for the radio that I had securely clipped to my ski jacket and radioed for help. And just before it got really cold and breathing became difficult, my colleagues found me.

I always worry about cancer and I have no wish to die, but I won't stop loving life and challenges. My story begins being caught in avalanche, the probability of which should be really low. I was young then, panicked that I would not survive, that no one would find me, that I would die all alone.

But my story took another turn and became one about

living—not dying—despite having fears and having cancer. And often the fears that haunt us are those that we think we cannot face but somehow do. I have had the privilege of accompanying so many amazing patients through my practice. I have seen joy, love, and desperation, but what is most striking are those moments when we recognize that no matter what, we can handle adversity and live beyond our fears.

For a long time, I was terrified of getting cancer again, lying awake at night, going to pieces from fear of having cancer when I have a pain somewhere. I am no longer afraid, just prepared. And in the meantime, I will appreciate what I have and am thankful for all the moments I can learn from, for my ability to do research, and for having spent time with amazing people— and even to hold their hands in a difficult moment.

And who knows what will happen next?

—Pamela N. Munster, May 2018

Acknowledgments

This story has been told in the hope that fewer and fewer patients will have to undergo the fates of my grandmother, my father, and myself, and with the thought that more awareness and early intervention can spare partners and friends, daughters and sons, sisters and brothers, mothers and fathers, from dying of cancer or undergoing serious surgery. In the future, no one should be the unsuspecting victim of a devastating illness like my father and so many others, or suffer the consequences of overlooked hereditary cancer.

So many dear friends, colleagues, and patients have shaped my outlook on life as a woman, physician-scientist—and ultimately patient—that the list would possibly be longer than this book. Some are mentioned in the pages you just read, and every day I am filled with the warmth of knowing all of them: the friends and colleagues who have helped me thrive with their gentle smiles, encouraging hugs, and profound confidence.

I work with the most creative and dedicated health care professionals, scientists and physicians both, without whose tireless and often all-too-underappreciated efforts, the advances

I so gratefully benefitted from would not exist. Words cannot completely express the connection a patient has with a health care provider, one that is both profoundly deep and perforce often distant. Thank you to the many providers and coworkers who have been part of my recovery, the many experts who let me ask them for advice, the many shoulders that appeared for me to cry on when I needed to most. Thank you to all the flight attendants who discreetly brought me a cookie when I sat by the window with tears flowing down my cheeks, during treatment, and when reliving those memories while working on this book, so I could hold it together when we landed.

I could not have gone through the year of therapy and continued seeing patients without the steadfast patience of my research team, who kept our work going, and all the clinical coordinators, nurses, and nurse practitioners who would always step in when I needed a minute.

I would like to express my deep gratitude to all the patients and families who are and those who are not mentioned in this book for their trust, and for the privilege to allow me to contribute to their care. I am richer for the time I spent with you. Some of their names have been changed, and some details of their stories slightly altered, to respect their privacy.

Profound appreciation and friendship goes to Linda Hudson Perigo, who in one conversation managed to encourage me to take on the task of telling this story, and then with expertise and guidance let me fall in love with writing. Only ever a phone call away, she has been instrumental in shaping the structure of the story, and through many long conversations and edits held my hand in bringing it to life. Thank you to my agent, Al

Zuckerman, for his support and belief in me. I truly appreciate the gentleness and kind guidance of my editor, Jennifer Kurdyla, who with true mastery shaped and rounded out my voice.

Profound thanks for my friend Emily Bergsland, who through my illness and the writing spent hours running with me through the forest guiding me through my treatments, sharing my fears, my hopes, and ultimately listening to me talk about this work while our lungs were on fire.

To the early readers of the book who have guided me with provocative questions on the purpose and details of this story: I could not wish for better friends than those who keep the bar high with love and kindness.

Deepest gratitude for my father, Norbert, for his courage and poise through a most difficult disease, for being a rock and guide throughout my life in sickness and in health, and for trusting me enough to guide him through his cancer. Profound love and gratitude to Marietta, who unwaveringly has been by his side and mine.

About the Author

Pamela N. Munster, MD, is a professor of medicine at the University of California, San Francisco, where she is leader of the Developmental Therapeutics Program/Helen Diller Family Comprehensive Cancer Center, director of Early Phase Clinical Trials Unit, and coleader of the Center for BRCA Research. In addition to her laboratory research, she focuses on developing novel strategies to treat patients with incurable cancers as an oncologist. She serves on multiple local, national, and international committees focused on developing new treatments for cancer, has published over two hundred articles, authored textbooks, and is a frequent lecturer. A native of Switzerland, she leads breast awareness campaigns in the US, UAE, and India.